Enlighten Your Path:
The Aspiring Yoga Instructor's Guide to
Mastering Teacher Training

Contents

Preface

"In the middle of difficulty lies opportunity." -Albert Einstein

Embarking on a Journey of Enlightenment

As Albert Einstein wisely illustrated, challenges present us with unique opportunities for growth, a sentiment at the core of our shared journey into the art of yoga instruction. This book unfolds as a guide and companion for those who have embarked on the transformative path to becoming yoga teachers. Within these pages, I hope to offer a structured yet tender exploration of the myriad aspects involved in teacher training—from the poetic rhythm of Sanskrit to the intricate dance of anatomy, and the delicate art of guiding a class.

My decision to write this book was driven by the recognition that many aspiring yoga instructors grapple with layers of apprehension. They are individuals who have both experienced the profound impact of yoga and are now yearning to share this gift. Yet, the journey ahead seems daunting. The fear of inadequacy looms large—fear of not understanding the ancient language of yoga, of not grasping the fine details of the human body, or of not engaging students effectively.

Throughout my years of experience, I've encountered numerous students—let's think of them as friends on a similar path. One friend, Jamie, confided that despite their passion for yoga, the thought of standing in front of a class filled them with dread. Another friend, Alex, was concerned about memorizing the Sanskrit names for poses and understanding the musculoskeletal nuances relevant to a safe practice. These conversations were heart-opening. They revealed not only the common threads of doubt but also the burning desire to overcome them.

These shared experiences, coupled with my own journey from apprehension to empowerment, led me to write this book. Consider it a beacon of hope and a tool for navigating the sometimes turbulent, often exhilarating waters of becoming a yoga teacher.

Inspired by the wisdom of countless yoga masters, the guidance of my own teachers, and the spirited conversations with fellow yoga enthusiasts, this book is woven from a fabric of collective experience, academic insight, and personal epiphanies. My heartfelt thanks go out to all who have contributed to this journey, either by sharing their vulnerabilities, offering their knowledge, or simply being a part of the vibrant yoga community.

To our dear readers, your decision to invest your time and attention in this guide is a courageous step toward realizing your dream. I am honored to accompany you on this path. **This book is crafted for those with a fervent passion for yoga and a budding aspiration to guide others through their practices.** No matter the level of familiarity with the academic or practical elements of teaching, what's indispensable is a willingness to learn, to grow, and to embrace your potential.

As we turn the pages together, imagine we are embarking on a journey where each step is aimed at enriching your understanding, boosting your confidence, and preparing you to step into the role of a yoga instructor with grace and poise. *You will emerge more knowledgeable, assured, and ready to transform not only your own life but the lives of those you teach.*

Thank you for granting me the privilege of guiding you through this journey. Let's together light the path to a future where your passion for yoga blossoms into the power to enlighten others. Continue reading, and find solace in knowing that the solutions you seek are just a few breaths away.

1

The Humble Yogi or Yogini's Ascent

The studio smelled of sandalwood and sage, a scent that somehow always managed to calm her. Maya's students were in Savasana, the room silent except for the rhythmic hum of deep breathing—a symphony of tranquility. She moved with grace between the mats, her gaze soft but keen, her mind, however, spoke in boisterous whispers. These moments of stillness often invited Maya to dance with her insecurities, ones she concealed behind a serene facade. She was their teacher, but was she not also a student? Her journey through the depths of yoga seemed to stretch before her like the vast, untamed ocean, each wave a lesson she had yet to learn.

Outside, the clamor of the city was awakening as the orange canvas of dawn slowly brightened into day. The transformation of the sky mirrored her own aspirations. Like the sky could not hold back morning's arrival, she could not cease to grow. Her practice was an endless climb, magnificent peaks conquered just to see another on the horizon. But doubts, like clouds, often obscured the warmth of progress. Was she enough for them? Did her imperfections at the front of the class belittle the wisdom she sought to impart?

As the class stirred from their final resting pose, Maya's fears knotted together in her chest, imposing and stubborn.

With every "Namaste," she felt the twine loosen, the collective energy of the room quelling her uncertainties. Her eyes met nods of gratitude—their silent accolades chipping away at the walls harboring her trepidations.

Later, when the last student had left and the quiet hum of the studio buzzed in her ears, Maya unfurled her own mat. Each movement was an intimate conversation with her insecurities; each stretch, a deliberate step toward personal enlightenment. The solitary practice was her harbor, where she whispered to herself the truths of her journey—continuous, unbound by the destination.

The day waned, and evening wrapped the city in its cool blanket. Maya sat alone, legs crossed, palms resting on her knees, and she breathed. Each inhalation was potential; each exhalation, a release of doubt. In the twilight of the empty studio, she found the courage to face her journey—one not marked by mastery, but colored by the honesty of continual learning.

What fears might you let go to step true on your path, where vulnerability is not weakness, but the foundation of strength?

Cast Aside the Cloak of Expertise

You stand at the threshold of a journey both ancient and enduring—each step upon this path adds a stone to the mosaic of your mastery as a yoga teacher. Picture the greatest yoga instructors of our time; they are perpetual students themselves, consistently exploring the vastness of yoga. True mastery is not found in a static state of knowing all, but rather in the unending adventure of learning and growth. As an aspiring yogi or yogini, it's imperative to internalize that the landscape of yoga is one of undulating hills, not insurmountable peaks, and your ascension is fueled by **humility and the courage to embrace the unknown.**

In this foundational chapter, **we pivot our gaze from the summit to the climb itself,** recognizing that the way upwards is non-linear, paved with both triumphs and challenges. Every master was once a beginner, and every yogi's journey is uniquely their own. As you stand ready to share your practice, let go of the notion that you must first conquer an Everest of knowledge. Instead, understand the strength in admitting what you have yet to learn. This admission does not undermine your abilities but instead showcases a remarkable strength of character indispensable to an inspiring instructor.

The Mirror of Learning Reflects Infinitely

Consider the reflective surface of a tranquil lake—it's the ancient mirror that yogis have gazed upon, seeking wisdom. You, too, are invited to look deeply and discern the contours of your ongoing development. Acknowledging that **yoga mastery is a lifelong pursuit** reminds us that there is no finality to what we can absorb. Our practices, our bodies, and our teaching methodologies all evolve—embracing this evolution is a commitment to an ever-expanding repertoire of knowledge and experience that enriches both student and teacher.

Acceptance Illuminates the Path

Many yoga instructors have grappled with feelings of inadequacy, where the myth of total expertise looms like a shadow over their confidence. To break free from these shackles, **embrace humility** as a source of light, guiding you through the mist of doubt. Summon the bravery to acknowledge your limitations, for in doing so, you carve out space for growth and new understanding. This not only ennobles your teaching practice but also nurtures an authentic connection with your students, who find solace in your shared humanity.

Feeling under-equipped is a natural part of the teaching experience, yet it is through this lens of self-compassion and **openness to new experiences** that great instructors are shaped. With each class you lead, each interaction with a student, and each hour of personal practice, you accumulate invaluable layers of insight. Transform the anxiety of 'not knowing enough' into an invigorating drive for learning, and watch as your teaching practice flourishes in response.

Strategies for Lifelong Cultivation

So, how does one actively cultivate this ongoing journey of improvement? Implement strategies that place personal growth at the heart of your teaching. Journal your experiences, seek mentoring from seasoned instructors, and expose yourself to a variety of yoga styles. Enhance your skill set through workshops and retreats, and let the vibrancy of the global yoga community stimulate your curiosity and passion. **Integrate continuous learning into your pedagogy** by sharing new insights with your students and inviting them to embark on their personal quests for knowledge alongside you.

In teaching yoga, the ultimate guide is your own practice—frequently return to it as both a sanctuary and a laboratory, where questions can be pondered and answers explored through movement and meditation. By embracing this process, you not only deepen your competence but also cultivate inner tranquility that radiates to every corner of your existence, and consequently, your teaching.

In the chapters ahead, you will delve deeper into the tools and philosophies that make an *enlightened path* accessible. Together, we will explore the fabric of Yoga Teacher Training, weave together the threads of anatomy, philosophy, and teaching methodologies, and provide strategies for crafting the tapestry of a fulfilling teaching career—all the while keeping your wellness and balance as primary wefts in this intricate work.

Remember, **each moment of learning is a step upwards on your ascent**—not toward an unattainable peak, but toward a higher version of yourself, as a teacher and as a seeker on the immutable path of yoga.

Acknowledging the Lifelong Journey

The ancient practice of yoga is more than a sequence of asanas; it's akin to an ever-growing tree. Just as a tree sheds old leaves to make way for new growth, yoga practitioners shed past limits as they learn and develop. The concept of mastery in yoga is not defined by the endpoint but by the journey itself, a perpetual expansion of knowledge and experience.

Imagine stepping onto your mat for the first time. Each posture, each breath, brings a sense of discovery. This novice state is where all yoga masters begin. It's essential to remember that even those revered gurus were once beginners themselves, learning the subtle intricacies of their bodies and the depth of their minds through yoga. The humility gained from acknowledging one's perpetual student status can become a foundation of one's practice.

A common misconception is that yoga mastery equates to flawlessly executing advanced poses. However, the heart of yoga beats in the rhythm of continuous exploration and growth. It doesn't demand perfection but rather commitment to the ongoing process of learning. Mastery is not signified by the final pose; it's championed every time an individual returns to the mat with a mindset to delve deeper.

In this journey, the analogy of a river can be insightful. A river does not cease to flow once it has traveled a certain distance; it continues, adapting to the contours of the land, forever shaping and being shaped by its environment. Similarly, as a yogi or yogini, one continues to flow through the landscape of yoga, learning new forms, and adapting to the teachings with grace and resilience.

The key understanding is that yoga mastery is not a destination, but a trek of endless learning.

Embracing Humility and Openness

In your pursuit to teach yoga, you might find the whispers of inadequacy echoing in your mind. But consider this: the most profound lessons often rise from the simple act of acknowledging that you do not know everything. The beauty of teaching yoga lies in the partnership between learning and instructing. Welcome the opportunity for growth; each class is a canvas on which both the instructor and the students paint new paths of understanding.

Humility in teaching does not signify weakness, but strength. It's the strength to admit when you are unsure and the courage to discover the answers alongside your students. In doing so, you not only deepen your own practice but also invite a genuine connection with those you guide. The shared experience of learning fosters a community where growth is collective.

Feeling inadequate at times is a human condition, not a reflection of your ability to teach yoga. Every class you lead offers a new experience, a chance to learn something about yoga, about your students, and importantly, about yourself. Replace feelings of inadequacy with a humble curiosity, and you open the doors to experiences that enrich your teaching and your soul.

Leaning into the discomfort of the unknown can be likened to approaching a challenging asana. Initially, there is hesitation, uncertainty, and a glimpse of fear. Yet, with repeated practice comes familiarity, ease, and ultimately, the confidence to approach even more complex poses. In teaching, this analogy holds true; familiarize yourself with the discomfort of the unknown, and let each experience hone your ability to guide others with assurance and poise.

What if, instead of fearing inadequacy, you embrace it as a signal to learn and grow?

Strategies for Continuous Learning

To ensure continuous development as a yoga instructor, one strategy is essential: embrace a beginner's mind, no matter your level of expertise. Entering each teaching session or learning opportunity with openness and curiosity keeps the passion for yoga alive. It allows for fresh insights, even into the most familiar practices, and maintains the spirit of discovery that attracted many to yoga initially.

Incorporating feedback is another crucial step. After each class, seek constructive criticism from students or mentors and reflect on it with an open heart. This feedback is invaluable as it helps refine your teaching methods and intensifies your understanding of yoga's impact on others. By actively listening, you demonstrate your commitment to personal and professional growth.

Consider also forming a community with fellow yoga instructors. Shared wisdom is a treasure trove of insights and support. Together, explore new aspects of yoga, discuss challenges, and celebrate triumphs. The collective wisdom of a community invariably strengthens individual members, fostering a supportive environment for learning and growth.

A successful strategy might involve setting specific goals for your yoga practice and teaching. Whether it's mastering a new set of postures, learning about yoga philosophy, or incorporating different teaching methods, clear objectives provide direction and motivation. Break down these goals into achievable steps that you can integrate into your daily or weekly routines.

By adopting strategies that cultivate personal improvement and integrating continuous learning into your pedagogy, you intertwine the core values of yoga with your teaching philosophy, honoring the journey, the humility, and the perpetual growth that define the ascent of the humble yogi or yogini.

Embrace the Journey Ahead

As you embark on this enlightening journey into the world of yoga instruction, remember, this is just the beginning. **Mastery in yoga teaching is not a destination to reach swiftly but a path to walk with humility and openness.** The belief that one must be an all-knowing sage before stepping into the role of a teacher can lead to self-doubt and insecurity. Instead, **understand that growth in yoga is continual, and each step forward is a stepping stone towards improvement**.

The Key to Success

The key to success lies in acknowledging that learning in yoga is a perpetual journey. Cultivating a mindset of perpetual learning will not only benefit you as a teacher but will also enhance the experience for your students. By **embracing the process of continuous improvement**, you not only enrich your practice but also inspire others on their own paths.

Nurturing Growth

As you move forward on this path, remember that **the journey of mastery in yoga is a blend of personal growth and professional development**. Embrace each new experience, each challenge, as an opportunity to expand your knowledge and refine your skills. By employing strategies that foster personal improvement, you will integrate continuous learning into your teaching practice seamlessly. Through dedication, openness, and a willingness to learn, you will **nurture growth within yourself and your students**, creating a harmonious environment for all.

    With the foundation laid in this chapter, exciting benefits await you as you delve deeper into the wisdom and intricacies of yoga instruction. Stay tuned to uncover more insights, techniques, and wisdom in the upcoming chapters that will empower you on your journey to becoming a confident and skilled yoga instructor.

2

The Language of Yoga: Beyond Sanskrit

Maya adjusted her tunic before stepping onto the wooden floors of the studio, the scent of incense and the muffled sound of a harmonium greeting her. She found her place, rolled out the mat with a quiet thud, and settled into a cross-legged seat, her eyes falling closed as her students filed in. Today, she pondered, would be different. She was a yoga instructor, not as fluent in Sanskrit as the ancient sages, yet she harbored a love for the soul of the practice.

A shaft of gentle sunlight broke through the window, falling across her face, a reminder that the sun salutes the earth every day without fail. Maya opened her eyes, the dancing dust particles in the beam of light seemed to encourage her to integrate that same dedication into her teaching - infusing it with Sanskrit, slowly, like the patient rise of dawn.

The class began, and the room filled with the symphony of deep breaths. Maya uttered the word "Asana", her voice a soft timbre among the quietude. She remembered how the ripples of the word seemed to mystify when she first heard it. Now, it flowed from her lips as naturally as the breath from their lungs. She watched the wave of recognition on her students' faces – they understood. Communication was her tool, Sanskrit a delicate instrument she was learning to play.

In the space between asanas, her mind wandered back to her teacher, Anand, whose voice resonated with the depth of the ocean whenever he spoke Sanskrit. She hadn't inherited that depth - not yet. But her heart beat with the rhythm of the practice, and that, she resolved, was enough.

As the session unfolded, like the petals of a lotus at dawn, Maya interwove Sanskrit terms with their English names. Her speech held the purity of spring water, clear and unassuming. She glanced at the faces before her, diverse, eager, connected not by language, but by the shared pursuit of balance.

The class reached its end, each student lying back into Savasana. Maya's voice drifted over them, a feather on the breeze, as she guided their relaxation. Her own heart relaxed with them - there was no barrier here, no right or wrong in the words she chose. The essence was in the experience.

She sat there, her fingers gently brushing the mat, the tranquil hum of the harmonium fading into stillness. She knew her journey with Sanskrit would grow, as all things do, with time and love. Maybe one day the words would sit as comfortably on her tongue as her body did in these poses. But until then, what was the deeper connection she was nurturing here, beyond the words and language?

Unraveling the Mysteries of Yoga Communication

When embarking on the journey from yoga enthusiast to professional instructor, one encounters a multitude of challenges and learning curves. Among these is the impression that a deep knowledge of *Sanskrit* is a gatekeeper to becoming a proficient yoga teacher. **Yet, it is not the fluency in Sanskrit that defines the quality of teaching but the ability to connect and communicate with students.** This chapter peels back the layers of language used in yoga, presenting a refreshing perspective for aspiring instructors: Sanskrit familiarity is beneficial but not mandatory for teaching effectively.

Yoga is a practice steeped in ancient tradition, and Sanskrit terms are undeniably intertwined with its essence. Understanding these terms can bring a sense of authenticity to your classes and deepen your own appreciation of the practice. **However, the focus of a successful yoga session is the experience you create for your students.** Any instructor's main priority should be to facilitate a safe, inclusive, and engaging environment. This starts with clear and accessible language that students of all levels can understand. Recognizing the importance of simplicity in instruction is the first step to effective teaching.

As an instructor, you'll find that **essential Sanskrit terms naturally weave their way into your lexicon.** Start by identifying these key terms and incorporating them slowly, fostering a learning atmosphere that welcomes curiosity without overwhelming your pupils. It's crucial to strike a balance where Sanskrit enhances rather than eclipses the teaching moment. Students should leave class feeling enriched with knowledge, not perplexed by jargon.

Seamlessly Weaving Language with Practice

Learning Sanskrit is akin to learning any new language; it's an evolving process. Initially, it might seem daunting, but repetition and practice will embed these terms into your memory. **Demonstrate through actions** as much as by words, allowing students to make associations between movement and language. They will begin to recognize asanas (postures) and pranayamas (breath control) not just by name but by the sensations and benefits they impart. This sensorial learning translates into a deeper comprehension that supersedes linguistic barriers.

Encouraging student participation is another technique to deepen language comprehension. Foster an environment where students feel comfortable repeating Sanskrit terms, asking questions, and even correcting their pronunciations. It's this collaborative learning approach that not only demystifies Sanskrit but also strengthens the community aspect of yoga class.

Inevitably, mistakes will happen, both on the part of the instructor and the students, but they are an integral part of the learning process. **Embrace the mishaps** just as you would encourage students to accept their physical limitations on the mat. This promotes a growth mindset – an indispensable tool not just in yoga, but in all facets of life.

Cultivating a Language of Inclusivity

Regardless of your proficiency in Sanskrit, the hallmark of an effective instructor is the ability to cultivate a language of inclusivity. Shift your focus from linguistic perfection towards cultivating a genuine connection. *Engagement, empathy, and attentiveness* are what your students will remember and appreciate. Be attuned to their needs, and be adaptable in your teaching methods. Different classes may require varying degrees of Sanskrit based on the familiarity and preferences of students.

Lastly, remember that as a yoga instructor, you are not merely a conduit of physical postures and breathwork techniques. **You are a guide on the path of mindfulness and self-discovery**, a role that transcends spoken language. Sanskrit can be an enriching addition to this journey, but it is your passion, knowledge, and dedication to your students that will leave an indelible mark on their yoga practice.

Embrace the gradual integration of Sanskrit at your pace and let your authentic teaching style shine. Your journey as a yoga instructor is not just about adopting a new vocabulary, but about crafting holistic and transformative experiences for your students – and this is an art form where heart and clarity speak louder than the perfect utterance of ancient terms.

Essential Sanskrit: A Tool, Not a Barrier

To step onto the mat as a teacher is to accept the responsibility of guiding others through their yoga experience. Sanskrit, with its deep-rooted place in the history of yoga, can add a layer of richness to this experience. Yet, knowing every Sanskrit term is akin to wanting every color of paint before starting a canvas. Not necessary. A few essential hues can create a masterpiece. It's vital to identify key Sanskrit terms that correspond to common poses, concepts, and practices, such as 'Asana' for posture or 'Pranayama' for breath control.

In this ocean of ancient vocabulary, remember that Sanskrit is but a single current. Your role as an instructor is marked by the clarity and accessibility of your teachings, not by the fluency of your Sanskrit. Envision someone learning to swim; they first need to grasp the basics of breathing and movement, not the technical terms describing each stroke. Incorporating essential Sanskrit terms should serve as buoys aiding navigation, not as anchors dragging down comprehension.

A thoughtful selection of Sanskrit terms introduced alongside their English equivalents bridges traditions without befuddling your students. Imagine you're planting a garden in which you wish both exotic and native plants to flourish side by side. By sowing seeds of understanding with clear explanations, your students can appreciate both the beauty of the language and the essence of the practice.

Nurturing this garden requires patience. Sprinkling your instruction with Sanskrit gradually integrates these terms into the shared vocabulary of the class. Keep explanations simple and context-driven, offering insights into the meaning and significance of each term. This way, the language unfolds naturally, like a lotus blooming in slow motion.

Embrace Sanskrit as a complement, not a prerequisite, to effective teaching.

Communication: The Heart of Instruction

Clear communication is the lifeblood of yoga instruction; it is the conduit through which the essence of practice is transmitted. Like a potter shapes clay into form, use words to shape understanding and guide experience. The goal is not to mold Sanskrit scholars but to cultivate proficient yogis. Instruction that prioritizes clarity over complexity empowers students to connect deeply with their practice.

Reflect for a moment on the tune of a well-loved song. Even if the lyrics slip away, the melody remains, resonant and true. This is the role of effective communication in yoga. It's not about the precision of Sanskrit pronunciation, but the harmony and rhythm of your instruction that resonate with the students. Your words, tone, and cadence—these are the notes that compose a memorable and transformative yoga session.

It's easy to assume that Sanskrit proficiency represents authenticity in teaching. Yet, authenticity emerges from the ability to be present and responsive to your class. When your focus shifts from reciting perfect terms to creating an inclusive and understandable practice space, you allow room for individual interpretation and growth—like a storyteller who speaks directly to the heart of the audience, weaving tales in a language that transcends words.

Use questions to prompt discovery, employ analogy sparingly to light up complex concepts, and never underestimate the power of demonstration. Offering a visual or tactile understanding can often communicate more than the most accurate Sanskrit term. After all, yoga is an experience first and a linguistic endeavor second.

Consider a guide leading explorers through a vast landscape. Does the guide overwhelm them with jargon and technical names for every plant and landmark, or prioritize keeping them engaged and confident in their journey? Strive to be a guide who illuminates the path, not one who shadows it with unnecessary complexity.

How might your words become the bridge that carries your students toward the heart of their own yoga experience?

Growing With Sanskrit

With each class you teach, your comfort with Sanskrit will naturally evolve. Discovering methods to seamlessly infuse this ancient tongue into your teachings can be compared to learning a musical instrument. Initially, you might struggle with the mechanics, but over time, as you play more, the music flows intuitively. Begin where you are, with the terms that feel most relevant and accessible, and let your repertoire expand organically.

Integrating Sanskrit can be as simple as associating terms with their meanings in real-time practice. For Asana names, pair the Sanskrit with a demonstration of the pose. This links language to action, creating a dual reference for visual and auditory learners. Like seasoning enhances a dish, let Sanskrit enhance the flavor of the experience without overwhelming the senses.

Create opportunities for repetition and reinforcement. Repeat Sanskrit terms gently during your sessions, and contextualize them within the fabric of the practice. This technique allows Sanskrit to become a soft echo in the background of your teaching, rather than a foreign sound demanding attention. Imagine adding drops of dye to water; gradually, the color permeates, changing the essence without immediately shifting the form.

Celebrate progress in language acquisition as part of the yoga journey—a journey of both body and mind. As you and your students advance, the use of Sanskrit serves not merely as a means of communication but as a nod to the lineage and philosophy of yoga. It becomes a gentle whisper of ancient wisdom that enhances the modern practice.

Integration of Sanskrit into your teachings is a journey of small steps leading to the grand tapestry of yoga instruction.

In embracing Sanskrit without being bound by it, prioritizing clear communication, and incorporating language with grace, you forge a teaching style that

is as effective as it is adaptable.

Keep It Simple and Effective

Remember, **Sanskrit familiarity is a bonus, not a barrier**. The essence of yoga lies in your ability to connect with your students, not in reciting complex Sanskrit terms flawlessly. *Focus on clear communication and building a strong rapport with your class.* Your students are here to learn, grow, and find inner peace through your guidance. By prioritizing their understanding and comfort, you create a nurturing environment where yoga can truly work its magic.

Practice Makes Perfect

As you delve deeper into your teaching journey, integrating Sanskrit will become more natural. Just like mastering any new skill, it takes time, practice, and patience. *Allow yourself the space to grow and evolve.* With each class you teach, you'll find yourself effortlessly incorporating Sanskrit terms into your instructions, enhancing the yoga experience without overwhelming your students. Embrace the process and trust in your ability to adapt and learn along the way.

Embrace the Journey

Your evolution as a yoga instructor is a beautiful journey of self-discovery and transformation. *Embrace each step along the way.* Let go of the pressure to be perfect and instead focus on being present, compassionate, and authentic in your teaching. As you immerse yourself in the world of yoga, Sanskrit will naturally weave its way into your vocabulary, adding depth and richness to your classes.

A Bright Future Awaits

With a solid foundation in place, you are well on your way to becoming an inspiring and impactful yoga instructor. **Re-

member, it's not about perfection, but about connection. Your passion for yoga and your dedication to helping others will shine through, guiding your students on their own path to self-discovery and wellness. Embrace the journey ahead with an open heart and an open mind, and watch as your teaching skills blossom and grow beyond measure.

3

Anatomy for Yogis and Yoginis: Safety First

The studio was silent but for the muted shuffle of feet on hardwood. It was a small room, lined with pale blue mats like neat rows of empty beds. Morning light, crisp and unyielding, flooded the space through tall windows. He stood at the front, Jake, a man who once staggered under the weight of his own body, now a pillar in this sanctuary. Today, he would teach for the first time.

His mind drifted back to the accident—a tumble down a flight of stairs that shook his life like a snow globe. Bones had mended, scars had faded, yet fear had made a quieter recovery within his chest. In his journey to heal, yoga beckoned—a dance of movement and stillness where he found his strength.

As the students entered, he observed each one—a tapestry of stories written in posture and gait. There was an unspoken kinship among them, one he now had to guide. They did not know of his sleepless nights spent poring over anatomy books, studying each sinew, each tendon, or his intimate dialogues with doctors who marveled at his recovery. His knowledge was the lamplight by which he would keep them safe.

Through the opening sequence, his voice was the quiet rumble of certainty. He watched the alignments like a seasoned sailor reading the stars, his eyes catching a knee angled too sharply, a spine curving where it should not. Adjustments were made, softly, as he remembered his own body relearning its symphony.

Late into the session, a middle-aged woman paused, gripping her knee. Jake's heart missed a beat; injury and its shadow were all too familiar tenants. He moved to her side, his mind a quick archive of potential ailments and remedies. "Breathe," he said, a single word to tether her to the moment. Guiding her through a modification, he felt the tide of worry subside within them both. They were passengers on the same voyage, seeking balance between strength and surrender.

He closed the class with a message of gratitude and growth, his own pulse still echoing the soft fray of nerves. As his students rolled their mats and carried the day's lesson with them, Jake was left with the echo of their movements and the scent of sweat and wood. He knew this was merely the beginning, his teaching a living entity that would grow with each life it touched.

For now, he was their custodian—the keeper of a practice that bore his scars and shared his triumphs. But how would his experiences—past and present—shape the way he'd nurture his students' journeys in the unfurling tapestry of anatomy and alignment?

Unveiling the Human Blueprint: A Yogi's Guide to Anatomical Wisdom

As an aspiring yoga instructor, you've likely experienced firsthand the profound impact of yoga on both body and mind. But beneath the surface of each asana, beneath every mindful breath, lies a complex network of bones, muscles, and tissues that are the silent partners in every yoga practice. As you turn the page to this vital chapter, prepare to bridge the gap between the ancient art of yoga and the scientific world of anatomy. Knowing your way around the human body isn't just an academic exercise—it's the cornerstone of **safe and**

effective yoga instruction.

The journey of an aspiring yoga instructor is riddled with challenges and discoveries, and one of the most critical revelations comes from the study of anatomy. It's a subject that can seem daunting at first, but the rewards are immeasurable. **Grasping basic anatomical principles** shields your students from injury, empowering them to practice with confidence. With every pose you instruct, you'll learn to see beyond the mat—to the skeletal cues, the muscular feedback, and the breath that orchestrates it all.

Whether you're guiding a seasoned practitioner into a challenging inversion or helping a beginner find comfort in a basic stretch, knowledge of **alignment, injury prevention, and body mechanics** is instrumental. Your cues and hands-on adjustments won't just enhance the experience; they'll act as a subtle language of care, **preventing harm** and promoting well-being. This doesn't require you to be a medical expert. Instead, focus on the essentials that tie directly into yoga's functional movement.

As you step into the role of both student and teacher, **developing strategies to expand your knowledge** becomes just as important as the initial learning itself. Your growth in anatomical wisdom will mirror the progress of your students; as they advance, so too must your understanding. The commitment to never-ending learning isn't a burden—it's a gift that keeps giving, preparing you to face every teaching moment with assurance and depth.

Remember, teaching yoga is as much about imparting wisdom as it is about creating a *safe sanctuary* for exploration and growth. **Your dedication to learning anatomy** is a testament to your commitment to your students' safety and a reflection of the respect you hold for the practice of yoga.

The Scaffold of Support: Step by Step to Anatomical Mastery

Understanding the Basics of Anatomy

- Take your first step into the world of anatomy by getting comfortable with the major players: the skeletal, muscular, and respiratory systems. Recognize how these systems come alive during yoga.

- Next, delve into the language that describes our body's infrastructure. Anatomical terms will become your tools for clear and effective communication.

- With the objective of protecting your students, explore the *alignment of yoga poses* and their impacts. Notice where vulnerabilities lie and how to fortify against potential strains.

Incorporating Anatomy into Your Yoga Instruction

- Start simple. Introduce anatomical basics to your students in a way that's digestible. **Visual aids and plain language** can bridge the gap between complex concepts and intuitive understanding.

- Emphasize the marriage of anatomy and safety. Teach the art of *listening to the body*, and encourage modifications as a form of self-respect and care.

- Guide with precision, using verbal cues and adjustments to shape the ideal alignment. Clarify that this isn't about achieving a picture-perfect pose—it's about **preventing injury** and enhancing the flow of energy.

Expand Your Anatomical Knowledge

- Commit to ongoing learning by seeking out additional resources like workshops and online courses specialized in yoga anatomy. Make this a scheduled part of your journey, allowing for both structured study and flexibility.

- Literature and research will keep your knowledge fresh. Regularly reading new publications will ensure you're up-to-date with the latest anatomical insights related to yoga.

- *Challenge yourself* by teaching students with diverse anatomical needs. This practical application cements knowledge and hones your adaptive skills as an instructor.

Integrate Anatomy into Class Planning and Sequencing

- When crafting your classes, wield your anatomical knowledge thoughtfully. Reflect on how each pose will engage the body, and tailor your sequences with anatomical intelligence.

- Use your class time to sprinkle in nuggets of anatomical wisdom. Frame it in a context that promotes **body aware-ness and appreciation**, and let students connect with their practice on a deeper level.

- Visuals are powerful teaching tools. Make use of charts or models to make anatomy tangible, illustrating the relevance to the practice at hand.

Reflect and Evolve

- Continual reflection is vital. Assess how you've woven anatomy into your teachings and seek feedback to improve.

- Keep curiosity burning. Attend discussions, network with peers, and never shy away from opportunities to expand your understanding.

- As your knowledge unfolds, let your teaching morph with it. Share this journey with your students, inviting them to redistribute their weight, realign their posture, and rediscover their practice through an anatomical lens.

This pathway to anatomical mastery isn't a one-way street; it's an *ongoing dialogue* between you, your students, and the ever-expanding world of anatomical knowledge. Embrace each step with the enthusiasm of a beginner and the wisdom of a sage, and watch as the safety and richness of your yoga classes flourish under your tutelage.

The Skeletal Framework of Understanding

Grasping the basic principles of anatomy, much like understanding the foundation of a house, is essential for ensuring the structure is sound. When we consider the anatomy of the body, we start with the skeleton, a rigid framework that supports and shapes the form, similar to how a scaffold shapes a building. This frame is the starting point for all movement and functionality within the body, bearing the load of our physical forms.

Just as architects must know the stress points and load-bearing capacity of a structure, you, as a future yoga instructor, need to comprehend where the body can flex and where it must remain firm. Knowing the map of bones and joints will help you see when a student's body deviates from safe alignment. Also, understanding which parts of the body are prone to injury allows you to guide students with caution, preventing unnecessary strain on vulnerable areas like the lower back or the knees.

Think of your learning as a gardener who begins with the foundational roots. The roots, akin to our bones, need to be nurtured with knowledge so that the practice of yoga blossoms safely in your classroom. Your role is to water these roots with clear instructions and watchful guidance.

Each bone, each joint, plays a specific role, just as every beam and pillar in a building has a purpose. You do not need to memorize every bone, but you should understand the major players like the spine, pelvis, knees, and shoulders. Recognize that each poses a specific path for stability and mobility, and it's within these paths that you will guide your students.

Understanding your students' anatomical frameworks is the cornerstone of their safety and successful practice.

The Blueprint for Balanced Practice

The Anatomy of Alignment   Understanding basic anatomy is like holding the blueprint for a harmonious building; it lets you spot the potential for imbalance or injury in a yoga practice. Focusing on alignment is like ensuring that the beams and columns of a building are in the right place to sustain the structure. Misalignment might not lead to immediate injury, just as a building doesn't collapse at once, but over time, the wear can lead to serious damage.

Step 1: Understanding the Basics of Anatomy

Taking your first architectural class, you would start with the basics—earthquake-resistant design, perhaps, or the types of materials that can withstand various stresses. In a yoga context, this starting point is learning about the skeletal, muscular, and respiratory systems, and how these systems underpin every yoga pose. Spend time familiarizing yourself with how these systems function both independently and as a unit during practice. Understand anatomical terms to communicate nuances with others.

Knowing the structure of common yoga poses is your first step to being an excellent instructor. Analyze these as you would a building's design, understanding where strain might occur or support might be needed, preventing situations where a student might, metaphorically speaking, 'buckle under pressure'.

Step 2: Incorporating Anatomy into Your Yoga Instruction

As a teacher, your job begins with translating complex architectural designs—in our case, anatomical knowledge— into simple sketches that anyone can understand. Simplify the language when you speak to your class about their bodies, using visual aids as necessary. Highlight the importance of alignment for injury prevention and efficient energy flows, in the same way a building's design affects its sustainability and comfort for those inside.

Use verbal cues and hands-on adjustments meticulously. Think of it like gently shifting a column into its proper place, to prevent future collapse and instead promote structural integrity within the body.

Step 3: Expand Your Anatomical Knowledge

Don't stop learning once you've passed your first few 'architecture' exams. Deepen your understanding by taking specialized courses in anatomy for yoga, reading up on new research, and staying abreast of developments. Practicing with those who have unique anatomical concerns can enhance your experience, much like an architect takes on projects with unique challenges to grow in their field.

Step 4: Integrate Anatomy into Class Planning and Sequencing

Just as an architect wouldn't haphazardly place a window or door, you shouldn't randomly assemble a class sequence. Consider the anatomical implications of each pose and how it will serve your students' bodies. During classes, offer anatomical insights that help students connect with their bodies, using visual aids like charts or models to enhance comprehension.

Step 5: Reflect and Evolve

Finally, keep refining your 'blueprints'—your class plans and anatomical explanations. Solicit feedback and stay curious, exposing yourself to a variety of anatomical perspectives. As your expertise grows, let your teachings evolve and encourage your students to explore their anatomies in innovative ways.

Could your refined understanding of anatomy be the blueprint for your students' breakthroughs in yoga practice?

The Living Anatomy of Yoga

While learning anatomy can be as dry as reading a technical manual, applying it to yoga breathes life into both knowledge and practice. Think of it as understanding a musical instrument; you may know what each part does, but to create music, you must learn how to harmonize them beautifully. This is analogous to how yoga harmonizes our breath (wind instrument), muscles (the strings), and bones (the structure of the instrument itself).

Step 1: Understanding the Basics of Anatomy

Your anatomy class has begun, and now it's time to delve deep. Like attic treasures discovered in an old house, you unearth the marvels of the human body. Initially, concentrate on how the major body systems—the skeletal, muscular, and respiratory—cooperate to perform yoga poses. Like a conductor learns the roles of different instruments in an orchestra, master the anatomical terminology to effectively guide your yoga symphony.

As you examine yoga postures, think about which 'notes' should be harmonious and which dissonant, identifying alignment and areas susceptible to injury.

Step 2: Incorporating Anatomy into Your Yoga Instruction

Armed with newfound knowledge, you're ready to compose your first simple chord progressions, or yoga flows, for your students. Introduce anatomical concepts in layman's terms, showing them the meaning of each pose and guiding them toward safe practice. Teach them how to listen to their bodies, to stop when they hear a 'wrong note' indicative of pain or discomfort.

Hands-on adjustments and verbal cues are your way of tuning the strings, ensuring a harmonic pose that resonates with health and injury prevention.

Step 3: Expand Your Anatomical Knowledge

Taking master classes in anatomy for yoga is akin to learning advanced composition techniques that elevate your teachings. Stay updated with the current trends in the field to enrich your knowledge. Encourage teaching students with various physical conditions, adding complexity to your compositions and fostering adaptability and empathy in your teaching style.

Step 4: Integrate Anatomy into Class Planning and Sequencing

Orchestrate your sequences with anatomical precision to protect and enhance your students' practice. Weave short discussions of anatomy into your classes as you would thematic variations into a symphony, enriching the overall experience and promoting bodily awareness.

Step 5: Reflect and Evolve

Always remain a student of the anatomy symphony; practice, invite feedback, learn, and adjust. Continue to infuse your classes with fresh insights from the evolving landscape of anatomical research. Adapt and grow as a teacher, and witness how your students become attuned to the beautiful music of their anatomically aligned yoga practice.

By intertwining teaching experiences with anatomical knowledge, you compose a symphony of safe, enlightened yoga practice for all.

Empower Your Teaching with Anatomical Knowledge

Now that you've delved into the vital realm of anatomy for yoga practitioners, you hold in your hands a precious tool for nurturing safe and fulfilling yoga experiences. **Grasping the basic principles of anatomy is not a mere step in your journey; it's the very foundation on which your teaching stands.** Remember, safety always comes first in yoga. Your understanding of alignment, injury prevention, and body mechanics is what separates a competent instructor from an exceptional one.

Elevate Your Instruction with Alignment Awareness

Alignment is the cornerstone of a fruitful yoga practice. It affects everything - from the efficacy of a pose to preventing potential injuries. Just like a finely-tuned instrument playing harmonious melodies, correct alignment orchestrates a seamless flow of energy throughout the body. Pay attention to alignment cues, guide your students with precision, and witness their practice bloom under your attentive eye.

Cultivate Wisdom through Continued Learning

Your journey as a yoga instructor is one of perpetual growth. **As you teach, always remain a student of anatomy.** Look for learning opportunities, attend workshops, and seek guidance from seasoned practitioners. With each class, each student, you'll deepen your understanding and refine your skills. Remember, a true master never ceases to expand their knowledge.

Embrace the Path Ahead

As you lock the treasures of anatomical wisdom within your teaching repertoire, you step into a new realm of possibilities. Your dedication to safety, alignment, and ongoing learning will not only set you apart as a proficient teacher but also as a compassionate guardian of your students' well-being. **Stay curious, stay diligent, and let the universe of anatomy unfold its secrets before you**.

4

The Art of Authentic Instruction

A lone figure, clothed in the quiet shades of twilight, sat cross-legged on the worn wooden floor of an old gymnasium now serving as a makeshift yoga studio. Around her, the soft hum of a settling building mingled with distant traffic, forming a cocoon of urban calm. Her name was Mira, a yoga teacher known for the light she carried within her, a light she hoped to ignite in others.

Her thoughts churned, a swirling river of anticipation and anxiety. A fresh-faced cohort of students would file in within the hour, each carrying their own invisible weights. In their eyes, she would seek the silent plea for a space that welcomed them as they were—broken, hopeful, human.

Yesterday's session lingered in her mind. She saw the student in the back, his brow furrowed, struggling not with the shape of his body but with the shape of his belief, his place in the world. Mira knew that what she offered in these classes stretched beyond the reach of her arms or the bend of her back. It was the authenticity she wove into her guidance, the permission she gave for everyone to stumble, to waver, yet to be strong.

A breeze drifted through an open window, carrying the scent of jasmine and the murmur of leaves. It embraced

Mira gently, as if to whisper, "Your passion is the beacon; let it shine." Embers of excitement flickered within her as she imagined the ways she could inspire growth and healing. She envisioned the safety she would create, a sanctuary amidst chaos where vulnerability was not just accepted but honored.

With each breath, she anchored herself to the present, a fortress of serenity amidst the torrent of her responsibilities. How could she carve out a space for self-discovery in this room that echoed with the echoes of basketball games and scuffed sneakers?

The sharp clack of the gym clock, as it marked the relentless march of time, pulled her back to her purpose. Mira unfurled her legs, palms pressed to the floor, as she rose to prepare for her arrival of her students. She wondered how each one might manifest their unique story in the language of limbs and breath. The notion warmed her, fueling her resolve to guide them not just through poses, but through the intricacies of their inner landscapes.

Would they understand that her teachings were mean to be seeds, planted with hope to flourish in the depth of their beings?

Discover the Heart of Teaching Yoga

Yoga, at its essence, is an experiential journey—one that's personal yet shared within the communal energy of a class. As an aspiring yoga instructor, mastering the technicalities of asanas and the theory of the ancient texts is just the surface. The real depth lies in **breathing life into your lessons** through authenticity and passion. You are not just teaching yoga; you are imparting an experience that could potentially transform lives.

Crafting a Genuine Learning Space

The creation of a genuine and safe learning environment begins with **trust and respect**. But how does one cultivate such an atmosphere in the yoga class? It starts with being present—truly present—for your students. It's the act of listening and observing, then responding with intuition and care to their needs. The spaces we occupy are filled with energies; as an instructor, your role is significant in shaping these energies into a supportive, non-judgmental sanctuary where everyone is welcome to explore and grow.

Infusing your classes with authenticity isn't simply about being relatable; it's ensuring that every word and motion resonates with the truth of your experiences and understanding of yoga. It's allowing your unique passion for the practice to spill into your teachings, whether you're joyfully demonstrating a sequence or sharing an insight from your personal meditation practice. Remember, students can sense when your heart is in your teaching, and this sincerity serves as a beacon for their own exploration into yoga.

Embracing Your Teaching Style

In yoga, as in life, authenticity is about embracing your unique colors. It's a dynamic interplay of your strengths, quirks, and the individual philosophy you bring to the mat. Encouraging student growth and self-discovery doesn't require you to have all the answers. Rather, it calls for you to be a gentle guide, who shows the way by *lighting the path with your passion* and allowing students to find their footing. This chapter will delve into the nuances of identifying and nurturing your teaching style—a style that is not imitated but cultivated through self-reflection and sincere connection with your inner teacher.

The Power of Vulnerability

To be vulnerable is to be powerful. In the context of leading a yoga class, it means having the courage to show up as you are—imperfections included. This vulnerability creates a subtle bond with your students, a shared human experience that builds the foundation for deeper learning. It's about swapping the pursuit of perfection for the grace of evolution, both for you and for those you guide. This chapter guides you through the strength found in vulnerability and how to let it elevate your teaching to new, more authentic heights.

When your presence in the classroom is **anchored in authenticity**, students not only learn yoga; they embark on their personal journeys with the freedom to be their true selves. It's an unfolding that you, as the instructor, get to witness and nurture, making teaching yoga an art form unto itself. Here, we will explore the artistry of authentic instruction. Not just the 'how', but the 'why'—why authenticity in teaching yoga isn't merely effective, it's essential.

Passion, the Seed of Inspiration

The enthusiasm you harness for yoga is contagious. It's capable of sowing seeds of inspiration within your students that bloom into dedicated practice. Your passion—when expressed genuinely—can motivate and uplift, fostering an environment rich for the growth and exploration of yoga. This chapter will not just encourage you to find that passion but also offer tangible ways to integrate it into every aspect of your teaching. Because when passion meets purpose, we witness the beautiful unfolding of yoga's true magic.

Conclusion

This chapter is an invitation—a clarion call to step into the light of your true self and let that light guide your teaching journey. It's about recognizing the instructor's role as a cultivator of safe spaces, a beacon of authenticity, and a celebrant of individuality. Strap on your yoga mat and pack your most authentic self on this enlightening voyage to teacherhood. Teach not just from the mind, but from the heart, and watch as the seeds of your authenticity grow into a forest of yogic wonder within your students.

Identifying Genuine and Safe Learning Environments

In the world of yoga teaching, the heart of a nurturing session is the creation of a genuine and safe learning environment. This requires a delicate balance. Like a gardener who tends to their plants, providing sunlight and shade in just the right amounts, an instructor must ensure that every student feels seen, respected, and at ease. The elements of trust, non-judgment, clear communication, and physical safety form the bedrock upon which students can explore and grow in their practice.

Physical safety in yoga is not dissimilar to finding shelter during a storm. The yoga studio must be a refuge where the physical integrity of each student is a priority. From the suitable arrangement of mats to the knowledgeable adjustments by the instructor, these practical aspects are crucial. It includes careful observance of alignment, offering modifications for asanas, and maintaining awareness of students' comfort levels throughout the class.

Creating a non-judgmental space is akin to an open sky, limitless and accepting of all. Mindfulness in language, an inclusive approach to teaching diverse bodies, and honoring the individual journey of each student are the gentle winds that uplift and encourage everyone. This means leading with empathy, celebrating progress regardless of its magnitude, and fostering a community where comparison is replaced with camaraderie.

Clear communication serves as the roots that steady and nourish the yoga practice. It's not just about guiding through poses; it's the art of making each instruction accessible, understanding the rhythm of the class, and providing a dialogue that supports the mind-body connection. Ensuring that verbal cues are comprehensible, that they resonate on a deeper, more personal level—that is what allows students to flourish within their practice.

To truly unlock the power of yoga, we must first secure the foundation: a genuine and safe learning

environment for all who step onto the mat.

Infusing Authenticity and Passion into Yoga Classes

When teaching, authenticity is your signature—it's the stamp that sets apart an ordinary class from an unforgettable experience. Like a painter, each stroke of authenticity colors the canvas of the session with life and personal touch. Every breath, movement, and word should convey your unique connection with yoga. Remember, authenticity is the bridge between the teacher you are and the teacher you aspire to be.

Passion for yoga is infectious. It kindles a flame that can ignite the dormant enthusiasm of students. When woven into the fabric of your teaching, it transforms the practice from a series of postures to an immersive journey. It's through the zeal of your voice and the sparkle in your eyes that students begin to understand the profound impact of yoga beyond the mat.

Say goodbye to the notion of a 'perfect' yoga instructor. The idea of perfection can be as elusive as a mirage in the desert, distracting and disheartening. Instead, prioritize realness. It's in the moments you share your struggles and triumphs that you humanize the practice and draw students closer. Let them see themselves in you, and watch as the trust blooms.

By bringing your individual story to each session, you offer students a unique narrative course in yoga. Your journey, with its ups and downs, becomes a beacon, illuminating the path for others. Through tales of personal insights and breakthroughs, students are inspired to forge their paths, guided by the light of your experiences.

Cultivating the soil of your sessions with the seeds of your own passion and authenticity allows for a rich harvest of connection and inspiration.

What might change if you see yourself not just as a guide, but as a storyteller, sharing the epic of yoga through the voice of your soul?

Expressing Your Distinct Teaching Style

Every yoga instructor has a melody—a rhythm and flow to their teaching that is as unique as a fingerprint. Just as no two musicians will play a note exactly the same way, no two instructors will teach a pose identically. Embracing your distinct teaching style is the embodiment of authenticity and is essential for standing out in the symphony of yoga voices.

Knowledge and skill are important, they represent the instruments in an orchestra. But it's the style of play—the personal flair—that makes the music resonate with listeners. Your teaching style could be the warmth in your encouragement, the creativity in your sequencing, or the soothing timbre of your voice as you guide relaxation. It is these subtle, yet powerful, signatures that etch your teachings into the hearts and minds of your students.

Encouraging student growth is much like tending to a garden. *Just as each plant requires different amounts of sunlight and water to thrive, each student needs a personalized nurturing approach to blossom in their yoga journey.* Provide the support and space for self-discovery. Share your knowledge and wisdom, but also empower students to listen to their own bodies and intuition.

As instructors, we must remain students ourselves—always learning, adjusting, and evolving. By doing so, we set an example that yoga is a continuous journey, not a destination. It fosters an environment where self-improvement is celebrated, where each new insight is a stepping stone to a deeper understanding of oneself and the practice.

By intertwining the elements of a safe learning environment, authenticity with passion, and a signature teaching style, we pave the way for a transformative experience—for both the teacher and the students.

Cultivate Your Authentic Teaching Style

As you wrap up the elements of authentic instruction in your mind, remember that at the heart of effective teaching lies your unique teaching style. Your individuality is not a flaw but a strength that sets you apart as an instructor. **Infuse your classes with your passion for yoga; let it radiate through your instructions and movements.** Your enthusiasm will not only inspire your students but also create a positive and welcoming atmosphere in your classes. **Express your distinct teaching style with confidence**, knowing that it is your authenticity that will resonate with those you guide on their yoga journey.

Encourage Student Growth Through Self-Discovery

In the world of yoga, growth is not measured by physical perfection but by self-awareness and transformation. As you guide your students through their practice, **encourage them to explore, discover, and embrace their unique paths**. Foster an environment where they feel safe to challenge themselves, make mistakes, and learn from them. **Celebrate their progress, no matter how small, and inspire them to continue their journey of growth and self-discovery.** Remember, your role as a teacher is not just to instruct but to empower and uplift those you teach.

Embrace the Art of Yoga Instruction

Teaching yoga is an art form that requires skill, dedication, and most importantly, a genuine love for the practice. **Create a space where students feel seen, heard, and supported**. Cultivate your teaching style with authenticity, infuse your classes with passion, and encourage student growth through self-discovery. As you embrace the art of yoga instruction, remember that your role as a teacher goes beyond guiding postures; it is about guiding hearts, minds, and spirits towards a deeper connection with themselves and the practice.

5

A Symbiosis of Tradition and Innovation

Amid the bustling streets of Rishikesh, India, where the Ganges River flowed with the promise of cleansing and the air hummed with the chants of ancient wisdom, Maya felt the weight of tradition and the pull of modernity grasp her by the soul. She lived where yoga drew breath, where every corner spoke of asanas and every sunrise brought the faithful to stretch and seek enlightenment. Yet, amidst this tapestry of the ages, she faced a tumult of her own - finding her unique voice in teaching a practice as old as time itself.

The sun dipped below the peaks of the Himalayas, casting amber on the water as Maya perused her collection of dusty texts and laminated anatomy charts. The dichotomy played across her studio like a dance of shadows and light. Ancient scriptures whispered of yoga's profound spiritual journey, of its birth from the Vedas, and of its goal to unite the individual soul with the universal consciousness. Meanwhile, the robust diagrams of the human body spoke a modern dialect - of alignment, muscle engagement, and the biomechanics of each pose.

In the quiet that followed her class, Maya rolled up the mats with care, the echo of her students' labored breathing now only a memory in the empty room. They came for different reasons - some sought the physical benefits, others a reprieve from the rattle of their minds. They trusted her to guide them, and that trust weighed on her heart like an anchor, mooring her to a sense of responsibility as vast as the river itself.

Her mentor's words, spoken with a voice softened by time and wisdom, visited her in moments like these. "A teacher is both a gatekeeper and a bridge," he had said. "Balance the eternal with the fleeting, the sacred texts with the science of movement, and you will light a path true to the spirit of yoga." Yet, how could she stitch such disparate worlds into a seamless garment, one that would fit the diverse tapestry of souls that stepped through her door?

The night brought a cool whisper through the open windows as Maya sat cross-legged, her eyes closed in contemplation. She searched the silent murmur of her thoughts for answers, for that elusive equilibrium she yearned to offer her students. She wondered if the solution lay not just within the wisdom of sages or the precision of anatomists, but in the lived experience that flowed between them - a river of insight as continuous and ever-changing as the Ganges itself.

As the moon cast its silver glow upon her shelf of scriptures and anatomy books alike, she pondered the question that threaded through her doubts and her dreams: How does one carve a space for the soul in a practice shared by flesh and bone, by breath and thought? And where, among the hallowed echoes and the scientific truths, would her voice sing true?

The Harmonious Blend of Yesterday and Today

The landscape of yoga is as varied and expansive as the human experience itself—a tapestry woven from threads of ancient wisdom and splashes of contemporary innovation. As an aspiring yoga instructor, you stand on the precipice of shaping a teaching style that honors both the time-honored traditions and the creative modern practices. Yet, how does one navigate these seemingly disparate worlds? How can you—poised to lead—find the sweet spot that merges the richness of the past with the spirit of the present?

Understanding different yoga philosophies and teaching methodologies is like discovering the multiple layers of your own practice. It's not merely about adopting a stance; it's about **immersing yourself into a river of knowledge** that flows through millennia. You learn the ancient scripts, the Sutras that have guided practitioners for centuries, not to duplicate them, but to understand the core upon which yoga stands. Simultaneously, the modern, scientific approach beckons with its focus on anatomy, alignment, and evidence-based benefits. Each offers invaluable insights—your task is to weave them seamlessly into your personal tapestry of teaching.

To master your teaching equilibrium, explore the ancient with the same vigor as the new. Recognize that the practice that has transfused through generations has changed and adapted, just as it must in your hands. **The balance is dynamic**, not static—it shifts as the societies and bodies we cater to evolve. Forging your path requires an understanding that this equilibrium is not about compromise but about creating a synergy that enhances the practice holistically.

Formulating an integrated approach is akin to an artist blending colors on a palette—some hues taken from the roots of yoga, others from the blossoming branches of contemporary thought. Your ultimate goal is to paint a picture that resonates with your beliefs and addresses the needs of your students. It's about crafting a personal philosophy and technique that rings true to the core of yoga while being responsive to the world it exists in today.

Yet, how do you ensure your blend pays homage to tradition without being shackled by it or leaning towards innovation at the cost of depth? It starts with **active reflection**

and a keen understanding of the principles that underpin yoga. Build your teachings on the foundation of yogic tenets, yet remain open to the ways these can be translated into modern, relatable practices. It's not a diverging path but a confluence where the streams of old and new meet.

Remember, as you embark on this journey of discovery and integration, your role as a teacher is not merely to disseminate information; it is to encourage growth, foster understanding, and inspire transformation. The teachings of yoga are profound, and your delivery should be *a conduit for the essence of these teachings to flow.* In learning to honor both the ancient and the innovative, you don't just teach yoga; you breathe life into its timeless wisdom.

In the coming sections, let's delve deeper into embracing diversity in yoga philosophies, identifying the pillars of traditional practice, and integrating them with modern methodologies. Let's find the essence of what makes yoga a transformative force for both the self and the collective. After all, becoming an effective yoga teacher is not just about mastering asanas—it is about *bridging worlds* and *creating a cohesive narrative* for your students to live and practice by.

Explore and Understand Different Yoga Philosophies and Teaching Methodologies

The roots of yoga are embedded deep within the rich soil of ancient wisdom, drawing nourishment from millennia-old practices. Whether through the Sanskrit verses of the *Yoga Sutras* or the energizing postures seen in Vinyasa flows, there lies a spectrum of philosophies that form the backbone of yoga's diverse landscape. To comprehend this fully, one must peer into the assorted teachings of yoga that range from the classical paths known in traditional texts to the dynamic innovations in today's yoga studios.

Yoga philosophies, much like different types of soil, each provide a unique foundation from which the practice can grow and flourish. Some adhere strictly to the eight limbs outlined by Patanjali, emphasizing ethical precepts and meditation, while others infuse Bhakti's devotional aspects or integrate Tantric techniques to awaken dormant energies within. Exploring these diverse teachings is akin to a gardener understanding the nature of his soil; it is integral for growth and the eventual harvest of wisdom.

The teaching methodologies in yoga are as varied as the practice itself. With traditions that draw from ancient Indian culture to modern interpretations designed for the fast-paced contemporary world, each method offers something unique. While there may be no 'one-size-fits-all' approach, understanding the array of methodologies available – from Iyengar's precise alignment focus to the fluid sequences in Ashtanga – equips a budding yoga teacher with the tools to adapt and resonate with every student's needs.

To truly absorb the essence of these philosophies and methodologies, consider the metaphor of an artist selecting colors from a palette. As an aspiring yoga instructor, your palette is filled with shades of knowledge from various schools of thought. While one yoga style might offer the solemn gray tones of introspection and discipline, another presents the vibrant hues of joyful movement and community. Integrating these colors onto the canvas of your teaching allows the creation of a picture that is as authentic as it is transformative to those who witness it.

Understanding different yoga philosophies and methodologies provides the foundation for an enriched teaching practice, honoring both the tradition and individual expression.

Find Your Teaching Equilibrium

As the world of yoga evolves, the challenge often lies in finding your unique balance as a teacher, rather like a tightrope walker poised between two skyscrapers – one rooted in ancient tradition and the other soaring with contemporary innovation. Striking this equilibrium involves a deep understanding and thoughtful incorporation of historical practices and the integration of modern approaches that resonate with today's practitioners.

Where do the teachings of the *Bhagavad Gita* intersect with the principles of biomechanics in yoga? The answer might not be immediately clear, but as you delve deeper, you may discover that the warrior's discipline aligns beautifully with the precise knowledge of the human body. This combination of old and new strengthens the yoga teacher's repertoire, offering a more holistic and relatable practice to students.

Isn't it compelling to speculate on how the steep traditions of yoga can coexist with the improvisations of our modern era? Imagine a world where the reflective ecstasy of a yogi meditating by the Ganges can be mirrored in the focused breath of a student mastering a pose in a downtown studio. By merging the wisdom of yore with the scientific advancements of today, you craft an inclusive teaching philosophy that breaks down the barriers between the esoteric and the empirical.

On a practical level, this could translate to integrating mindfulness and meditation techniques from classical yoga into a fitness-oriented class structure. For instance, beginning a high-energy Vinyasa class with a few moments of intentional breathing can introduce a taste of mindfulness that deepens the experience beyond physical exertion.

When sowing the seeds of yoga tradition into the fertile ground of modern practice, it can result in a lush garden of options for students. With each asana, pranayama, or meditation technique you teach, there is an opportunity to cross-pollinate ancient wisdom with cutting-edge knowledge, creating a robust and adaptable yoga practice that caters to the individual yet respects the collective heritage.

Finding equilibrium as a teacher is like tuning a musical instrument; each string must resonate at the right frequency for harmony. As you tune your teaching to the diverse notes of tradition and innovation, consider what alignment feels most authentic and inspiring to you. Could it be that blending the millennia-old philosophies with current pedagogical methods is not just possible but beneficial?

How can the age-old wisdom of yoga enhance the current well-being trends and create a harmonious symphony within your teaching style?

Formulate an Integrated Approach

In constructing your teaching philosophy, consider it akin to building a bridge — a structure that connects the time-honored shores of yoga tradition with the bustling mainland of contemporary innovation. Your integrated approach should be both stable and versatile, capable of bearing the weight of history while adapting to the ever-changing landscape of the modern world.

Each asana practice, pranayama session, or meditation mindfulness can be seen as a brick in this bridge. With your understanding of different yoga philosophies and methodologies, you are now equipped to choose the materials that best represent your beliefs and serve your students' needs. The practice is no longer just about individual poses but about creating a cohesive experience that tells a story – your unique narrative as a teacher.

Would it not be truly profound, then, to build a yoga class that is more than just a physical workout but a journey through the layers of self that yoga philosophy unveils? Visualize weaving the threads of *Patanjali's Yoga Sutras* with a well-crafted asana sequence, inviting practitioners to explore the union of mind, body, and soul, thus enriching their understanding of yoga's depth.

Yet, it's important to note that the integration of these approaches should not be forced or inauthentic. Remember, the most enduring bridges are those that are designed with care and understanding of the landscapes they connect. As with any yogic endeavor, your teaching approach should remain responsive to the fluctuations of life, honoring the wisdom of the past while embracing the dynamic needs of the present.

Stepping beyond the role of instructor to that of a guide on this metaphorical bridge, you inspire your students to traverse from the familiar terrains of physical postures into the serene vistas of mindfulness and philosophy. Your compassion and insight inform your integrated approach, creating a nurturing environment for your students to grow.

In merging the old with the new, you forge a teaching path that is as authentic as it is engaging, as grounded as it is enlightening — encompassing the essence, diversity, and depth of yoga, while catering to the evolving spirit of your students.

Finding Your Balance

As you wrap up this chapter, it's clear that navigating the world of yoga philosophy and teaching methodologies is no easy feat. *Balancing tradition and innovation* requires a delicate touch, like holding a perfectly aligned yoga pose. Just as in yoga practice, finding that equilibrium between the roots of ancient wisdom and the branches of modern evolution is crucial for your growth as a yoga teacher.

Embracing Your Authenticity

Remember, at the heart of teaching lies your unique voice and perspective. **Embrace** the journey of self-discovery and let it **guide** you in formulating an integrated approach that truly reflects who you are. Your teaching style should not only resonate with your beliefs but also cater to the individual needs of your students. This personal touch is what will set you apart as an authentic and inspiring yoga instructor.

Striking a Harmonious Chord

In your quest to merge tradition and innovation, aim to create a synthesis that feels natural and balanced. Think of it as harmonizing different notes in a melodious tune. **Blend** the ancient wisdom of yoga with the contemporary tools and practices that speak to you. Find where the past meets the present in your teaching, creating a seamless flow that honors the roots of yoga while embracing the ever-evolving landscape of modernity.

Moving Forward with Confidence

As you move forward in your teacher training journey, remember that **finding your unique balance** is not a destination but a continuous exploration. Allow yourself to grow, evolve, and adapt as you delve deeper into the rich tapestry of yoga. Stay open to new ideas, techniques, and philosophies, while also honoring the timeless wisdom that has been passed down through generations.

In the next chapter, we will delve into the practical aspects of embodying your teachings and honing your skills. Prepare yourself to step onto the mat of knowledge with confidence and grace, knowing that your foundation is solid, your approach is authentic, and your journey is just beginning. Keep an open mind, a compassionate heart, and a steady breath, for the path ahead is illuminated by the light of your own inner wisdom.

6

Grounded in Practice: The Teacher's Path

In the gentle embrace of dawn, the sky held the promise of warmth yet delivered a brisk breeze that stirred the chimes hanging from the porch of a small cottage nestled in the heart of the countryside. Inside, Ana's bare feet kissed the cool wooden floor as she unrolled her yoga mat, a ritual as essential as the rising sun. With each posture, each breath, she sought the union of body and spirit, the same union she aimed to impart to her students.

The world outside fell away as she transitioned from Downward Dog into Warrior Pose. The clarity of her mind's eye was sharp, and in this focused gaze, she saw a reflection—a teacher not just demonstrating, but embodying the principles of yoga. The challenge was not simply in perfecting the asanas but in capturing their essence, threading it through her lessons like a subtle yet transformative undercurrent.

Her breath flowed in time with the whispering leaves that rustled in the wind beyond her window. Pranayama—the life force that invigorated her teachings with authenticity. Each inhale drew in inspiration from her surroundings, each exhale a release of stale doubts. She pondered the notion, how could the serenity she found in this practice resonate within the walls of her bustling classroom? The question stretched with her as she held her pose, steady and strong.

As she coiled into the grounding posture of Child's Pose, Ana savored the brief moment of repose. It reminded her that teaching was much like this—offering guidance and then stepping back, allowing room for growth. The wisdom she honed here on her mat was to be distributed like seeds among her students. Would they take root? Would this gift of self-practice bloom in their own lives?

The morning aged, and the sun climbed higher, casting light across her calm visage as she moved through a seated meditation, her mind a vessel filled with the deep waters of thought. She emerged with insights dancing like sunlight on the surface. What revelations from her journey on the mat could take seed in the hearts of those she guided? It was a question that beckoned her forward, a mantra woven through the fabric of her life's work. Could a personal revolution of the soul indeed be the catalyst for collective metamorphosis in the classroom?

Beyond Asanas: Cultivating the Teacher Within

When embracing the role of a yoga instructor, it's easy to fixate on the stretch of muscles and the alignment of limbs, but the heart of a truly remarkable teacher beats in time with their own practice. The whispers of wisdom in each breath taken, the silent strength in every asana held, this is where a teacher's journey begins. **Your personal practice is your compass, your mentor, and your muse**; it's the wellspring from which your unique teaching style will grow.

A sincere dedication to personal practice is the linchpin for professional growth as a yoga instructor. The mat is a canvas where *personal insights* emerge, painting the strokes of vulnerability and authenticity in your classes. When a teacher stands before their students, their practice does not simply inform their teaching — *it transforms it*. Through personal exploration, you discover the resonances of your own voice, crafting a symphony that speaks to the alignment of the body, the focus of the mind, and the liberation of the spirit.

The daily ritual of yoga practice deepens more than just one's physical flexibility; it cultivates a mental pliability that prepares you to face the myriad teaching moments with grace. Whether invoking the calm of meditation or the vigor of a powerful vinyasa flow, each personal session is a stepping stone towards a more fulfilled teaching experience. Imagine guiding your students not just through sequences, but through the same challenges and triumphs you've encountered on your mat — this shared journey is a potent catalyst for learning.

To be an instructor is not merely to demonstrate poses, but to impart a lived experience of yoga's transformative power. Through your own practice, you unearth the subtle art of awareness and the intricate mechanics of movement. You become attuned to the nuances of breath and the rhythms of stillness, which are essential threads in the tapestry of a yoga class.

Steps to Synthesis: The Harmony of Self-Practice and Teaching

Step 1: Establishing a Personal Yoga Practice

An earnest commitment to a rigorous and heartfelt practice begins with ordaining times of reverence on your yoga mat daily. The increment of duration is secondary to the consistency of this sacred ritual. Find or craft a space that beckons your presence, adorning it with simple yet significant tokens that speak to your spirit. Delve into the diverse expressions of yoga, from the gentleness of Hatha to the spirited dance of Ashtanga. Let joy and fulfillment be the yardsticks by which you measure the effectiveness of your chosen practices.

Step 2: Reflecting on the Benefits of Your Personal Practice

In the quiet aftermath of practice, sit with yourself, reflect on the ebb and flow of your internal energies. With each session, observe the subtle shifts, the incremental advancements in your body's dialogue with gravity, and your mind's dalliance with tranquility. Transcribe the journey of your practice into a journal; let it be a testament to your growing understanding and a mirror to reflect on the evolution of your practice. Embrace each session as an experiment, a playground where fear takes the backseat, allowing you to roam free in the realms of discovery.

Step 3: Integrating Personal Practice with Teaching

Carry the kernel of wisdom gathered from your personal practice into the heart of your teaching. Vulnerability shared is authenticity gained, and there is profound strength in revealing your growth and challenges to your students. Weave your favorite sequences or breathing techniques into the fabric of your classes, personalizing them with a passion that is uniquely yours. As you metamorphose as a teacher, let your practice be a mutable companion, adapting and expanding to reflect your pedagogical evolution.

Step 4: Exploring the Intersection of Practice and Teaching

Reflection becomes the bridge between your practice and teaching styles. Examine how personal insights inform your pedagogy, how the truths encountered on your mat can shine light on your students' paths. Trial and teaching go hand-in-hand; let your classroom be a crucible where your practice-fueled convictions are tested and refined. Actively seek out the reflections of your students, and use their feedback as the chisel to sculpt your instructional methodology.

Step 5: Cultivating Mindfulness and Self-Reflection

Beyond physical asanas, lay the foundation for a nurturing mindfulness practice. Embed contemplative sessions into the rhythm of your day, aligning them seamlessly with your asana practice. Engage in a dialogue with yourself, probing and contemplating your strengths and edges as an instructor, always through the lens of compassion. With each cycle of teaching, reaffirm your commitment to growth, treating successes as celebrations, and stumbling blocks as stepping stones.

In the realm of yoga teaching, personal practice is not a luxury; it is a necessity. **It is the invisible thread that weaves together the fabric of a class, the pulse that gives life to your teaching**, and the intimate conversation between you and yoga that every student hears and learns from, even in silence. In this chapter, as we explore ways to solidify and deepen this connection, remember that *your practice is the manuscript from which your teaching script is continually rewritten.*

Establishing Roots for Your Teaching Tree

Imagine your yoga practice as a grand tree with deep roots. Each daily session with your mat and meditation cushion drives the roots deeper, anchoring the towering structure of your teaching career. Your personal practice serves as nourishment, feeding each leaf and branch that reaches out to your students, allowing for a robust and blossoming presence as an instructor.

It's well established that a firm personal practice underlies the effectiveness of a good yoga teacher. Dedication to your own routine will enable you to speak from experience, empathize with your students' struggles, and offer genuine encouragement. A consistent practice brings an intimate understanding of asanas, breathwork, and meditation—essential tools for conveying the nuances of yoga to those you teach.

To distinguish between merely performing asanas and truly

engaging with them, consider the analogy of cooking. Anyone can follow a recipe, but a chef who tastefully seasons dishes has a palate refined by tasting a multitude of ingredients. Similarly, honing your palate in yoga—your sensory and experiential understanding—requires immersing yourself in regular practice.

Yet, not all practices will look the same, and what works for you may not be the best approach for another. Here lies the beauty of personal practice—it's a bespoke fit, tailored to your body, mind, and spirit, ready to be modified and perfected. Your practice is a laboratory where you are both the scientist and the subject, finding the perfect formula of techniques that you'll share with your students.

A dedicated personal practice enriches every aspect of teaching.

The Scaffold of Self-Enhancement: A Step-by-Step Process to Enrich Teaching

Step 1: Establishing a Personal Yoga Practice Begin by setting aside time each day for your yoga practice, even if it's brief at first. As your routine becomes a nonnegotiable part of your day, gradually expand your sessions to delve deeper into your practice. Create a space that resonates with tranquility and encouragement—your personal sanctuary where distractions fall away and focus prevails.

As you explore the asanas and the rhythms of your breath, recognize the many doors they open in terms of teaching methodologies. With every pose, there's a story of flexibility and strength; with every breath, a lesson in control and surrender. Your dedicated practice is your script, a narrative rich with insights ready to be translated into instructive gold for your students.

Step 2: Reflecting on the Benefits of Your Personal Practice In the same vein, reflection acts as a mirror to your soul. Post-practice, sit with the effects, the subtle shifts within your body and mind. A journal by your side can capture the essence of these transitions—a testament to your evolving practice and a wellspring for teaching inspiration.

Documenting your yoga journey is not just for memory's sake; it is an integral part of your growth as both practitioner and teacher. It is the silent witness to your discipline and self-discovery, charting a course you can share to guide others.

Step 3: Integrating Personal Practice with Teaching

Let the energy and authenticity of your personal practice seep into your classes, transforming them into an extension of your yoga journey. Your experience becomes a template, offering a structure yet allowing room for improvisation. As no one practice suits all, your work is to adapt and share the version that resonates with you, inviting others into a space that is uniquely enriched by your personal touch.

Step 4: Exploring the Intersection of Practice and Teaching

Keeping a pulse on the effectiveness of your teaching is crucial. How do your personal practice discoveries play out in your classes? Be the custodian of your methodology, but allow your students' feedback to shape the direction and refinement of your classes. Your teaching is a fluid expression of your personal practice, adapting in real time to the unfolding needs and revelations of both you and your students.

Step 5: Cultivating Mindfulness and Self-Reflection

A teacher's journey is paved with continuous self-reflection and an enduring commitment to growth. Mindfulness is an indispensable companion on this path, lending clarity to your introspection. Regularly taking stock of your teaching approach—its strengths and areas ripe for enhancement—ensures your practice's lessons are effectively transmitted to your students.

Developing a mindful approach to teaching lifts the veil on learning opportunities inherent in every class you lead.

What might change if you viewed every teaching moment as an extension of your personal mat?

Translating Personal Insight into Universal Wisdom

Your personal yoga journey is like a well of profound insights. With each practice, you draw nourishing wisdom from this well, and it becomes incumbent upon you to share this wealth with your students. As you transpose your experiential knowledge into lessons, imagine your teachings as water, flowing from the wellspring of your practice to the fertile minds of your students.

Step 1: Establishing a Personal Yoga Practice In nurturing this well, begin with the soil around it—your daily practice. It sets the rhythm of your days and cements the commitment to deepen the resonance of your teaching voice. Each session is a step towards a more robust understanding, a firmer grip on the tools necessary to lead others on their paths.

By embracing a variety of practices, you cultivate a broad seedbed of knowledge. As diverse seeds grow into different plants, so can your range of yoga exercises bloom into an eclectic teaching style.

Step 2: Reflecting on the Benefits of Your Personal Practice Reflection is the sunlight nourishing this growth, transforming physical movements into insights that transcend the mat—a metamorphosis of sorts. This reflection feeds back into your teaching, empowering you to lead students through their own processes of transformation.

A journal then becomes an invaluable chronicle of how to plant these seeds of practice within your students, capturing the ebb and flow of your yoga journey and shedding light on how those ripples affect others.

Step 3: Integrating Personal Practice with Teaching Each insight gleaned from your practice is a tool to build a bridge between personal growth and collective learning. Sharing these tools with students not only strengthens their practice but also forges a deeper connection, as they see their teacher in the trenches with them, working and evolving in parallel.

Step 4: Exploring the Intersection of Practice and Teaching As you refine your practice, it reflects in your methodology, becoming a living curriculum. Your resilience and adaptability as a yogi inform your teaching, guiding students to persevere in their practice just as you do in yours.

Drawing from your personal experience, you can craft an authentic narrative that resonates with those who have chosen to follow your guidance. Effective communication becomes the vessel through which your practice's learnings flow into the classroom.

Step 5: Cultivating Mindfulness and Self-Reflection Complete the cycle of growth with feedback—both internal and external. Ask yourself critical questions and welcome the observations of others. A teacher is a perpetual student, open to lessons from all quarters.

Embrace this exchange as an essential part of the teaching experience. Celebrate your strengths, acknowledge your shortcomings, and appreciate each step of your evolution. This journey, while personal, has the power to inspire a community of practitioners.

By intertwining personal practice, pedagogical reflection, and the translation of insights into teachings, fortify the bridge that connects your growth to that of your students.

Embracing the Journey

Establishing a consistent and dedicated personal yoga practice is not just about going through the motions on the mat; it's about cultivating a profound understanding and connection with the essence of yoga. **Your daily practice is where the magic happens.** It's where you refine your skills, deepen your knowledge, and tap into your wellspring of inspiration. As you dedicate yourself to your practice, you'll find that the benefits extend far beyond the physical postures. **Your practice becomes a mirror that reflects your growth, challenges, and insights.** It is through this commitment that you pave the way to becoming a truly impactful yoga instructor.

The Bridge to Teaching Excellence

Reflecting on how different aspects of your practice influence your teaching methods is like unraveling a beautiful tapestry of wisdom. Each asana, every breath in pranayama, and moment of stillness in meditation has a purpose that transcends the physical realm. **By dissecting and understanding these components, you gain a deeper insight into the art of teaching.** Your experiences on the mat become invaluable resources that shape your pedagogical approach. **Honor the lessons learned in your practice by infusing them into your teaching.** Your students will not only see but feel the authenticity and depth of your teachings.

The Ripple Effect

Translating the insights gained from your personal practice into valuable lessons for your students is the heart of effective yoga instruction. **Your practice is a reservoir of wisdom waiting to be shared.** As you guide your students through their practice, remember that you are not just leading a class; you are fostering a transformative experience for each individual. **Infuse your teachings with the pas-**

sion, understanding, and authenticity that stem from **your personal practice**. Let your journey inspire and uplift those who walk the path with you.

Cultivate Your Practice, Elevate Your Teaching

Nurturing your personal practice is not just a means to an end; it is the cornerstone of your journey as a yoga teacher. **Invest in yourself, commit to your practice, and watch as your teaching abilities flourish**. The more you immerse yourself in your practice, the more profound your impact will be on those who seek guidance on the mat. Embrace the transformation that comes from a dedicated practice, and let it illuminate your path as a beacon of light for others to follow.

7

The Grace in Every Misstep

Morning light filtered through the heavy foliage, casting a lattice of warm, golden beams onto the rustic wooden deck where Sam stood. He leaned over the wobbly banister, surveying the garden's overgrowth, considering the day's tasks ahead. His thoughts drifted to the mentoring program he volunteered for; tonight he would guide a group of eager, yet inexperienced, teachers.

The aroma of damp earth rose to meet him. He pulled his gaze from a butterfly navigating a cluster of daffodils, its journey a delicate dance of persistence and adaptation. Sam appreciated the metaphor in its flight; each glide and flap were a lesson in resilience. He knew well that in the art of teaching, he had been that butterfly, each mistake a gust of wind redirecting his course, each challenge a chance to refine his technique.

Inside, a stack of papers cluttered the corner of his desk, representing hours of efforts, reflections on what went well and what did not. Sam often lingered over them, ensuring he turned every error into a curriculum for improvement. As he sifted through his files, the phone trilled, startling a silence that had, for the moment, seemed complete. It was a reminder of the fleeting nature of tranquility in the life of one committed to the service of others.

This call, from a former student now a teacher herself, desperate for advice, put his personal plans in pause. She talked of her struggles to connect with her students, the lesson plans that fell flat. Sam listened, his heart tightening with empathy. He prescribed no instant remedy but instead shared his perspective on viewing these hurdles not as failures, but as fertile ground for growth.

As dusk pulled its shade over the sky, Sam reflected on the conversation. The sparkle of early stars accompanied a newfound silence. He pondered if his own counsel might be a light for others the way the stars guide travelers through the night. Would his mentee find solace in her own journey, recognizing each misstep as a beat in the rhythm of learning, much like he had found on his path? And who among us doesn't search the skies, wondering which of those distant lights will guide us home?

Embracing the Imperfect Journey

When we embark on the path of becoming a yoga instructor, we sign up for a journey of continuous learning and self-improvement. Our moments of triumph are often intertwined with challenges, and it's within these challenges that the deepest learning occurs. Recognize that the art of teaching is not only in the perfection of postures but **in the resilience we build from our teaching experiences**. Whether in a structured studio setting or a casual class with a group of friends, each opportunity to guide others through their practice propels us forward in our development.

Mindfulness is at the heart of yoga; it should also be the pulse of our instruction. Each class we lead is a new canvas, a tapestry woven with the threads of our words and gestures. There's an undeniable grace in every misstep because it provides us with a direct insight into where we can refine our skills. **Viewing every class as a laboratory** not only alleviates the pressure of striving for perfection but also establishes a fertile ground for growth.

The beginner's mind is a powerful one; it is curious, open, and untainted by the confines of 'getting it right.' As teachers, we must learn to **cultivate a beginner's mindset towards our own teaching practice**. When an instruction falls flat, or a sequence doesn't resonate as intended, instead of retreating into self-doubt, we must look at these instances as pivotal learning moments.

The Value of Diverse Teaching Scenarios

A common misconception is that teaching opportunities are limited to the time spent leading official classes. This narrow perspective can limit the scope of where and how we practice our craft. The aspiring yoga instructor should seize every chance to teach, be it in formal settings or impromptu sessions. These interactions are instrumental in refining one's teaching methodology and approach. *By embracing a variety of scenarios*, we open ourselves up to dealing with the unpredictable and adapting on the fly - an invaluable skill for any teacher.

Learning from the Uneven Path

In the tapestry of our teaching journey, mistakes are not just inevitable; they are the rich hues that add depth and character to our practice. Developing resilience is about responding constructively when faced with these moments. It's crucial to remember that *resilience is not inherent but honed over time*. With each class we teach, we get to practice bouncing back with grace and setting the stage for a better next class.

Imagine students as mirrors, reflecting back the clarity of our instructions and the effectiveness of our communication. It is through this reflection that we can objectively assess our teaching and determine where enhancements can be made. By **fostering a feedback-friendly environment**, we convert perceived obstacles into stepping stones, inching us ever closer to the epitome of the teacher we aspire to be.

Challenges as Opportunities

Rather than approaching challenges with trepidation, reframe them as opportunities. A challenging student, a difficult question, or a slip in sequence—each one is a golden ticket to a higher level of capability and confidence. *Embrace these occurrences as integral parts of your teaching narrative* and witness how each encounter enhances your instructional finesse.

In teaching, as in yoga, it's the journey, not the destination, that matters most. The path is winding, often looping back on itself, with each round providing a deeper understanding and stronger foundation. **There is grace in embracing every step of this journey**—the good and the difficult—as each experience enriches your ability to guide others with empathy, expertise, and genuine insight. Take heart in the knowledge that with each challenge comes a fresh chance to shine brighter, guiding both your students and yourself towards the serene transition to teacherhood.

Recognizing Teaching Opportunities for Skill Refinement

In the realm of yoga instruction, every moment spent guiding others is like planting a seed in the fertile soil of experience. Formal teaching engagements are akin to tended gardens, with structures and patterns, while informal sessions—perhaps with friends or family—resemble wild meadows, offering their own array of unexpected growth opportunities. Both environments are crucial for an aspiring yoga instructor's development, serving as living laboratories where skills can be honed and refined.

Consider the informal teaching moments as the unsung heroes of skill development. These understated scenarios, free from the pressure of formal student-teacher dynamics, provide a safe space to explore and expand your teaching style. Like a sculptor in the quiet of their studio, away from the prying eyes of critics, you can chip away at the raw marble of techniques, steadily revealing the form of your unique instructing voice.

Moreover, formal teaching opportunities come with a different set of expectations and benefits. They are more structured and typically involve a clear exchange, where the roles of teacher and student are well defined. In these sessions, feedback is often direct and measurable, leading to distinct areas for improvement. This feedback is the compass that guides the growth of your teaching capabilities; it helps navigate through strengths and weaknesses, shaping the course towards your full potential as an instructor.

To avoid the stagnation of your teaching abilities, grasp every chance to lead a class, no matter how small or informal the setting might be. Just as a river cuts through rock not by its power but by its persistence, your constant practice in a variety of teaching situations gradually carves out a master teacher from the novice within.

Every teaching opportunity, whether formal or informal, is an indispensable workshop for refining your yoga instruction skills.

Developing Resilience Through Mistakes

Mistakes are the silent teachers that often shout the loudest lessons. As an aspiring yoga instructor, you will find that each slip, each stumbled word, and each misaligned posture is not a setback but instead a cornerstone for building resilience. Learning to not just bounce back, but to bounce *forward* from these missteps is what cultivates the depth and flexibility required both in yoga postures and in teaching methodologies.

Have you ever noticed how a tree might bend in a strong wind, but rarely breaks? It's in this natural flexibility that the tree finds its strength. Similarly, when a mistake occurs during a class, it's an opportunity to model this adaptability to your students. Instead of dwelling on the error, gracefully acknowledging it and moving forward exemplifies a key yoga principle: presence and adaptation to the moment.

Acknowledging that mistakes are not mere obstacles but crucial parts of the learning process allows you to reconstruct the notion of perfection. Dispelling the myth of the flawless teacher is vital since striving for unreachable standards sets one up for perpetual dissatisfaction. Think of your teaching practice like clay in your hands, moldable and amendable. Even when misshapen, it can still be worked into something beautiful and functional.

The way to develop resilience is not through avoidance but through engagement with the possibility of mistakes. With this mindset, you will not crumble under the pressure of achieving perfection but rather embrace each class as an experiment where errors are expected and solutions are creatively sought. This acceptance transforms the soil of your teaching landscape, making it rich and conducive to growth.

Therefore, ask yourself: How do your missteps become the footprints that others might follow on their yoga journey? As they witness your recovery from errors, they learn the invaluable lesson that perfection is not the goal—continuous progress is.

By learning how to constructively respond to and correct mistakes, you build resilience that powers your growth as a yoga instructor.

Embracing Challenges as Opportunities for Growth

When stepping on the mat to teach, every challenge faced is like a new asana in your practice—a chance to deepen your understanding and enhance your balance. The advanced yoga poses are not there to highlight deficiencies but to usher in a new level of mastery over the body and mind. Similarly, teaching challenges, be they disengaged students or unexpected questions, are opportunities to extend your instructional prowess.

Just as a seasoned gardener knows that the hardest soil often yields the strongest plants, an aspiring yoga instructor understands that it's the toughest classes that grow their abilities the most. When you view a teaching challenge as a seed of opportunity, you shift your perspective from one of apprehension to one of potential. Every question that stumps you is a chance to learn something new, and every setback is a springboard for advancement.

Infusing this mindset into your teaching approach frames each class as a unique path toward becoming a more skilled and adaptable instructor. It demands a presence of mind and a willingness to see beyond the surface turbulence of a difficult situation. Embrace the idea that the more challenging the teaching experience, the richer the rewards in wisdom and skill.

A key step in this growth-oriented mindset is the reflection post-challenge. What lesson can be extracted? What new strategy or adjustment can be implemented next time? By conducting a mindful review after each class, the insights you gain multiply, cementing the lessons learned into your teaching repertoire.

View every teaching challenge as a vessel of growth, and your journey as an instructor will be marked by continuous expansion of your skills and wisdom.

The journey through missteps and challenges is not one to be shied away from but one to be welcomed with open arms. Through each informal practice session, each mistake made, and each obstacle overcome, the aspiring yoga instructor forges a path paved not just with success, but with the grace of growth and the richness that comes from learning.

Embrace Growth Through Teaching Opportunities

Engaging in teaching opportunities, whether they be formal or informal, is a crucial aspect of refining your skills as a yoga instructor. **Every moment spent guiding others through poses, breathing exercises, or meditation techniques is a chance to hone your craft**. These experiences not only help you become more comfortable in your role but also give you firsthand insights into what works well and what could be improved in your teaching approach.

Learn From Your Mistakes

Mistakes are not setbacks but rather stepping stones on the path to mastery. As you navigate through your teaching journey, there will undoubtedly be times when things don't go as planned. Instead of viewing these moments as failures, see them as opportunities for growth. **Each misstep is a lesson in disguise, teaching you how to handle challenges with grace and resilience**. Embrace your mistakes, learn from them, and watch how they transform into valuable teachings that sculpt you into a more skilled and adaptable instructor.

Cultivate a Growth Mindset

Shift your perspective to see every teaching challenge as a chance to enhance your skills. By viewing obstacles as opportunities for development rather than roadblocks, you pave the way for continuous improvement and evolution. **Embrace a growth mindset that thrives on challenges, welcomes feedback, and seeks out learning in every situation**. This approach not only propels your teaching abilities forward but also instills a sense of confidence and adaptability that sets you apart as a dedicated and resilient instructor.

In the world of yoga instruction, growth is not only about mastering poses; it's also about cultivating a teaching style that is authentic, empathetic, and responsive to the needs of your students. **Through teaching opportunities, learning from mistakes, and embracing challenges as avenues for growth, you are not just refining your skills as a yoga instructor but also nurturing a resilient spirit that will guide you on your path to becoming an inspiring and transformative teacher.**

8

In the Footsteps of Giants: Mentorship in Yoga

Arjun's feet moved with a steady rhythm, pressing into the warm mat that laid out on the chilled hardwood floor of the small studio. Windows fogged slightly from the early morning breath of the few steadfast students that followed his lead. His heart beat in tandem with the mantra softly playing in the background. Arjun had walked this path of a yoga instructor with careful steps, but recently, his stride had faltered.

This morning's class felt different, as if each motion was a question hanging in the air, unanswered. He observed his students, a mixture of earnest faces and limbs stretching towards personal growth, yet Arjun's own growth seemed to stagnate. "Am I offering enough?" he pondered, watching a particular student struggle into an imperfect warrior pose. His mind drifted, thinking of the teachers he admired, ones with decades of experience whose mere presence conveyed a depth of knowledge and confidence he yearned for.

The class flowed onwards, their movements a stream where Arjun felt like a stone caught between currents. The silent hum of the city outside crept in through the cracks in the old glass, whispering stories of countless souls in search of guidance. It mirrored the silent call in Arjun's chest—a beckoning to seek out a mentor. Each asana he guided his students through was meticulous, a silent testament to the practice, yet a reflection of his own quiet search for something greater.

In the cooling serenity of savasana, as his students lay with eyes closed and hearts open, Arjun stood still, an island of contemplation amidst a sea of tranquility. He thought about the ways he could strengthen his foundation, not just in yoga, but in his teachings. "Could I find a mentor who would understand, who would challenge and support me in the ways I need?" he asked himself with a hopeful trepidation. The room filled with the sound of collective breathing, a reminder that the path of learning is never trodden alone.

As students rolled up their mats, offering smiles and thanks, Arjun felt a spark of resolve. Today he would take the next step, reaching out to those teachers whose steps had once shaped the very mat he stood upon. The class dispersed into the bustle of the awakening world outside, each individual carrying a piece of the peace he had helped cultivate.

The studio now empty echoed with the faintest sounds of the city, symbolizing the myriad of lives each moving through their own narratives, encounters, and lessons. It was not just his students who were in a constant state of learning and growing; Arjun realized that this was his journey too. In seeking mentorship, maybe he would not just advance his own knowledge, but also pass on the flame of understanding to those who would walk the path after him.

Would a mentor see in him the potential he felt within? Could their wisdom be the key to unlocking the fullness of his own abilities as an instructor?

Standing on the Shoulders of Seasoned Yogi Masters

The path to mastering the art of yoga instruction is one filled with personal discovery, physical challenges, and pedagogical breakthroughs. But embarking on this journey solo can be as bewildering as attempting an advanced asana without proper grounding. This is where the value of mentorship—an often underappreciated asset in yoga teacher training—becomes crystal clear. Aligning yourself with a seasoned yoga mentor, someone who has navigated the winding paths of teaching, provides access to a reservoir of knowledge that can support you in leaping over hurdles in your training that might otherwise trip you up.

When discussing mentorship, **the emphasis lies on the relationship developed** with those experienced teachers who are pillars of wisdom. These are the individuals who have not only built their own practices from the ground up but have also helped others create their foundations. They can share lessons, insights, and provide the guidance needed to tailor your teaching style to the yoga mat. By unlocking the significance of these relationships, one begins to appreciate the nuanced complexities of guiding a yoga class and catering to a diverse group of students with varying needs.

Navigating Through Questions to Wisdom

Learning to ask pertinent questions is akin to mastering the breathing techniques that are an integral part of yoga—both require confidence, focus, and a sense of purpose. Through inquiry, a yoga trainee can elicit specific advice and insights that address their personal aspirations and challenges. *It's not merely about the answers received, but about developing the capacity to understand which questions will illuminate your path forward.* By probing your mentor's experiences, mistakes, and successes, you gain a multi-dimensional view of what it means to be a proficient yoga teacher.

A crucial aspect of mentorship is knowing that it's not a one-size-fits-all situation. Each mentorship relationship is as unique as a fingerprint, changing and evolving as you progress through your training. It requires attention, respect, and sometimes a bit of courage to delve into the depths of your mentor's experiences. In the delicate balance of listening and practice, there often lies a treasure trove of practical advice that can shape the way you overcome your own training obstacles.

The Confidence to Teach is Earned

Your teaching foundation and confidence as an instructor do not manifest overnight. Instead, they are the products of time, experience, and the supportive scaffolding provided by your mentors. Utilizing the guidance of a mentor is paramount in reinforcing the skills and self-assurance you need to stand in front of a class poised and ready to share the ancient practice of yoga. It involves embracing vulnerability, admitting what you don't know, and allowing yourself to be shaped by the hands of those who have already sculpted successful yoga practices of their own.

The journey to becoming a proficient yoga instructor is enriched immensely by the teachings of a mentor. It's a process that finely tunes your instructional abilities while fortifying your purpose and philosophy as a yogi. The chapters of your development as an instructor are co-authored by the mentors who lend their narratives to enhance your growth. **Their wisdom is not just spoken; it's a living practice,** demonstrated through how they encourage you to embrace your authentic teaching voice, supporting you in becoming not just an instructor, but a beacon within the yoga community.

In essence, mentorship in the realm of yoga is a sacred exchange that accelerates learning and nurtures professional development. It plays a critical role in not only enhancing your pedagogic techniques but also in elevating your entire approach to yoga as a practice and as a way of life. The legacy of great yoga teachers isn't found in the poses they perfected but in the students they inspired and cultivated to carry forth the torch of teaching. By seeking and valuing mentorship, you weave yourself into this noble lineage, ensuring that your journey transcends the physical and becomes a resounding contribution to the ever-expanding yoga universe.

Exploring the Significance of Seeking Mentorship

Mentorship in the field of yoga is as essential as the foundation on which a house is built. Without a solid foundation, even the mightiest of structures can falter. Similarly, without the wisdom imparted by experienced guides, an aspiring yoga teacher's practice may lack depth and understanding. These seasoned instructors, who have traversed their own paths of learning and teaching, become illuminating beacons. They guide through example, their insights akin to a lantern shining through the fog of our nascent experiences.

Imagine then, embarking on a hike through unfamiliar territory. The guidance of someone who knows every twist and turn of the path can make the journey not only easier but also more enriching. **In the world of yoga, established teachers act as these knowledgeable guides, leading the way through their mastery and insight.** By engaging with them, aspiring instructors gain clarity and perspective that only years of practice can bestow.

It's essential to recognize this relationship as a two-way street—a sacred exchange where respect and eagerness to learn meet the willingness to share and teach. In the context of yoga, this translates to not only perfecting asanas but also embodying the philosophy and ethics that come with the practice. Here, the idea of 'guru-shishya parampara', or the teacher-disciple tradition, comes into play, highlighting the age-old practice of passing down knowledge in an intimate and personal manner.

To seek a mentor is to make a conscious choice to grow, to acknowledge the gaps in one's knowledge, and to embrace the opportunity to fill them. By cultivating these relationships, an aspirant delves deeper into their role, understanding the nuanced layers of teaching yoga—beyond simply instructing poses, extending to inspiring transformation within their students. The significance of this cannot be overstated, as it is the very essence of what it means to teach yoga.

The key point: establishing a mentor-mentee relationship with experienced yoga teachers is pivotal to deepening one's understanding and practice.

Learning to Ask the Right Questions

When we reach out for mentorship, it's not just about receiving advice; it's about engaging in a dialogue where both parties learn and grow. To truly benefit from the knowledge of a mentor, one must master the art of inquiry. **Learning to ask the right questions is akin to learning to navigate a river; one must know when to paddle and when to let the current guide you.** Aspiring yoga instructors should seek to understand not only the how but also the why behind practices and philosophies.

Each question is a stepping stone toward greater understanding— a catalyst for revelation. It is a skill to discern which questions to ask that can unravel the complexities of a posture, the subtleties of breathwork, or the intricacies of meditation. **The mentor's answers can then weave a rich tapestry of knowledge that informs the practice on a deeper level.** Ask about their challenges, their triumphs, and the lessons that only experience can teach. This act of querying is as much a part of the learning process as the answers themselves.

But to extract the true value from this dialogue, one must also learn the art of listening. The answers may not always be direct; often, they lie between the lines, in stories, analogies, and even in the silence. Just as a seed needs the right environment to germinate, so does the wisdom from a mentor require open-mindedness and patience to take root.

When navigating one's own teaching hurdles, the experiences of a mentor can offer a much-needed perspective. Integration of their advice into one's training can transform challenges into teachable moments. **It's not about mimicry but about adaptation—taking the kernel of their wisdom and applying it to one's unique teaching style.**

If a question sparks an answer that lights up a new way of thinking, then the true power of mentorship is realized. **Mentors can often see the potential within us that we may overlook, and by asking the right questions, we harness their insight to not only grow as teachers but also as individuals.**

Could asking your mentor about their most profound moment of growth as a teacher lead you to your own?

Strengthening Your Teaching Foundation

Standing before a class, ready to impart knowledge, requires more than just understanding the mechanics of yoga—it requires confidence in one's ability to teach. **Mentorship serves as an invaluable scaffold that supports the development of a sturdy, reliable teaching foundation.** By consistently engaging with mentors, an instructor solidifies their skills and cultivates the self-assurance necessary to guide others.

Consider a tree, deeply rooted and towering skyward. Its strength doesn't come merely from its visible structure but from the unseen roots that anchor it firmly into the earth. In the realm of yoga instruction, mentors help nurture these roots, offering stability through shared experiences and support. They provide the nutrients of wisdom that allow an instructor's capacity and confidence to flourish.

Nurturing one's teaching foundation often involves recognizing and acknowledging one's vulnerabilities. A mentor not only points to the areas that need strengthening but also celebrates with you the growth that comes from confronting these challenges. Every insight, correction, and piece of advice is a brick laid down on the path to becoming a more resilient, knowledgeable, and empathetic instructor.

Rome wasn't built in a day, and neither is the confidence to stand in front of a class as a yoga teacher. It is forged in the moments of uncertainty, strengthened by the supportive words of a mentor, and cemented through practice and reflection. Utilize their feedback, observe their teaching methods, and soak in their approach to handling difficult situations. Through such engagement, the confidence that once seemed elusive begins to emanate naturally from within.

Confidence is the byproduct of mentorship—each discussion, each piece of advice, and each shared experience collectively heightens the instructor's sense of readiness. As your confidence grows, so does your ability to inspire and motivate students, to challenge them, and to cultivate a transformative space within your class. Mentorship, then, is not just about what you learn, but also about how you embody and convey that learning to others.

The culmination of seeking mentorship, asking incisive questions, and building a solid teaching foundation converges to a singular point—transformative growth as a yoga instructor, both personally and professionally.

Seeking mentorship from experienced yoga teachers is like having a guiding light in the vast world of teaching. **Connecting with these seasoned instructors can truly elevate your practice and teaching skills.** By absorbing their wisdom and guidance, you can navigate through the challenges of teacher training with more ease and confidence.

Absorb Wisdom and Ask Questions

Learning from mentors is a two-way street. **Ask the right questions to extract valuable insights and advice from them.** Don't be afraid to delve into their experiences and seek solutions to your training hurdles. Approach each lesson with an open mind and a thirst for knowledge.

Strengthen Your Teaching Foundation

Mentorship is not just about gathering information; it's about building a strong foundation for your teaching journey. **Utilize the support and expertise of your mentors to refine your skills and gain confidence in your abilities as an instructor.** Embrace their feedback and incorporate it into your practice to grow and excel in your teaching practice.

Embrace the opportunity to learn from those who have walked the path before you. **Mentorship in yoga is a powerful tool that can shape your teaching style and help you navigate the challenges of teacher training with grace and resilience.** So, step into the footsteps of giants, and let their guidance illuminate your path to becoming an enlightened yoga instructor.

9

Cultivating Confidence: Preparation Meets Authenticity

Kiran stood silently amidst the clamor of the bustling yoga studio. Mats unrolled like tongues, eager for the stories their owners' bodies would tell. The aroma of lavender and sandalwood wafted through the air, weaving a serene tapestry that briefly masked the pungent reality of human endeavor. Distinct conversations mingled into an indistinguishable hum; students chattered about their day, the usual prelude to the silence that yoga demands.

Today, Kiran faced an inner turmoil that mirrored the cacophony around them. They grappled with the weight of expectation, not from their yoga students, but from the one that peered back in the studio's mirror-lined wall. A class needed to be structured, a flow constructed that could carry the collective breath from the opening Om to the concluding silence. Kiran sought a sequence that would resonate deeply, knowing the true challenge lay not in the construction but in the delivery – for how does one mold the intangible? Preparation was the scaffold, but the capacity to be present, to adapt, stood as the building's architecture.

Thoughts drifted to last week's class and a frown caressed Kiran's brow. They recalled the rigidity of their instruction, the stiffness that stemmed from over-preparation. It was as if each asana was a rehearsed line in a play, leaving no room for the art of spontaneity. The memory taunted them – a stark reminder that the soul of a class was birthed in the unscripted moments between breaths.

Silently, Kiran retreated to a corner of the room and settled on their own mat, grounding themselves like the ancient banyan in their grandmother's tales. The knotted roots of these teachings whispered lessons of resilience, of connection, of authenticity. It was there, in the quiet recesses of their mind, that a decision took root – they would speak from the heart, let their true self guide the class. The thought was freeing, like a leaf finally surrendering to the autumn's call.

As their students began to settle, Kiran rose like dawn itself. The first rays of their smile warmed the expectant faces before them. They spoke, and their voice carried the calm certainty of the earth beneath them. With each breath-guided movement, there was a subtle acknowledgement of knowing and not knowing, of planning and letting go. Their gaze, soft yet penetrating, held each person, silently affirming that they too had a space within this woven circle of trust.

A hush fell over the room as they transitioned into Savasana, the death posture, a profound silence where the real yoga begins. In stillness, Kiran watched the rise and fall of chests, each one a testament to the life within. They reflected on how each interaction, each adjustment, bore the mark of their experiences, their very essence, and they wondered – could the sharing of one's own journey be the bridge that connects the wisdom of a tradition with the heartbeat of the present?

Holding the silence a moment longer, Kiran knew the question wasn't meant for them alone. How much of ourselves do we dare to weave into the tapestry of our teachings, and what magic awaits in the balance?

The Nexus of Knowledge and Intuition

Embarking on the path to becoming a yoga instructor is both an inner and outer journey. In this exploration of mastery, every instructor-to-be learns that confidence on the mat isn't inherited—it's cultivated. As you traverse the landscapes of teaching methodologies and personal discovery, remember that the essence of teaching yoga seamlessly blends preparation with the ineffable quality of authenticity. Imagine constructing a bridge between the worlds of meticulous planning and the freedom found in genuine self-expression. This bridge acts as the supportive structure that allows your students to journey towards their own understanding of yoga under your confident guidance.

Your first beacon illuminates in discovering **effective preparation techniques for structuring** and delivering classes that leave an impact – not just on the body but also on the soul. It's within these foundational plans where the seeds of a transformative class are sown. Yet, a truly adept teacher also knows the significance of balance, weaving together thorough class preparation with the supple thread of adaptability. Your documented plan must be as alive and breathing as the beings following it, able to bend and flex with the moment's call.

As the tapestry weaves further, it's an understanding that **integrating your true self** into teaching is what enkindles a palpable connection with your students. Authenticity cannot be feigned—and your students will feel a resonance when you speak and act from a place of sincerity. The yoga space becomes a canvas where your genuine passion for the practice paints inspiring and heartfelt strokes.

Let's delve into a process that encapsulates the facets of preparation, adaptability, and authenticity—a **Progressive Sequence of Empowerment** that lends you the clarity and the charisma to guide others through their yoga journey. Through this, the foregoing principles aren't just inscribed in your instructional manual; they become the very essence of your teaching philosophy.

Progressive Sequence of Empowerment

The goal of this process is straightforward: to create a yoga class that feels both solid in its structure and fluid in its delivery. The guided steps not only facilitate a well-organized session but also an enriched experience for both you and your students—one that honors where each person is in their individual practice.

Step 1: Preparing for Class Structure and Content

Dedicate time to outline the goals and objectives, giving your class a clear direction. Whether it's a journey through the chakras or a focus on strength and stability, let every choice be deliberate, from the poses you select to the words you utter. **Create a logical flow** that glides from warm-ups to more intense asanas, then gracefully descends into relaxation, much like a symphonic composition reaching its crescendo.

Developing your sequence is akin to writing a story—with a beginning that captivates, a middle that engages, and an end that provides closure and reflection. Place careful thought into each transition, making space for students of varying abilities by incorporating options and modifications that welcome everyone to your session.

Step 2: Creating Class Materials and Props

Visual aids and handouts crystallize your verbal instructions, reinforcing learning through multiple channels. Just as an artist selects their palette, **prepare your classroom props with intention.** Each tool should serve a purpose, enhancing your student's exploration of their practice. Arrange your space so that these items are not obstacles but stepping stones.

Step 3: Setting the Tone and Atmosphere

The initial moments in class are where the outside world dissolves, and the inner experience amplifies. Begin with a centering exercise, as simple as syncing with the breath, to establish a communal energy. **Create a serene ambiance** that supports your teaching intentions, remaining mindful of elements like lighting and temperature—factors that deeply influence the collective mood.

Step 4: Delivering Instructions and Cues

Your voice is the thread that guides students through the tapestry of their practice. Speak clearly, use concise language, and demonstrate when words fall short. Offer the gift of choice through variations, allowing each individual to respect their current physical state. **Teaching is an art of verbal sculpture**, shaping the empty space into a vessel of learning and experience.

Step 5: Being Present and Adaptable

While your lesson plan is a map to a destination, remember that the journey itself is where the true teaching unfolds. Observe and respond to the energy in the room. **Adaptability is the mark of a confident teacher**; it speaks of your ability to walk alongside your students, rather than leading from a distance. This step is fluid—it dances between structure and the spontaneous moments that arise when minds and hearts are open.

Evaluating the results emerges through reflection post-class. Consider the feedback, both verbal and observed in the body language and engagement of your students. Success in this context is the realization that both you and your students have grown through the process—where confidence as an instructor and the satisfaction of your class intertwine.

Remember, this is not a singular journey, but one that repeats with every class you lead. Each time you embark on this Progressive Sequence of Empowerment, you refine your skill, enhance your authenticity, and, most importantly, uplift your students.

Preparation Makes Perfect: Effective Class Structuring

A guiding principle for any yoga instructor is the art of preparation. We start by designing a yoga class sequence with clear, thoughtful progression. The blueprint of a well-prepared class fuses anatomical knowledge with mindful pacing, guiding students from grounding postures to invigorating peaks, and back to restful ease. It's a dance of movement and stillness aligned with the breath.

Imagine a garden where each plant requires a specific arrangement, sun, and soil to flourish. Constructing a yoga class can be likened to this gardening -- each pose or "plan" is carefully placed for optimum growth, rooted in the understanding of students' needs, much like plants in their varying environment. The garden's design reflects the gardener's knowledge and intention, with space and resources expertly allocated to create a thriving ecosystem.

Identifying the intentions behind each class is vital. Are we aiming to energize, relax, or deepen meditation practices? Each goal requires corresponding elements—a dynamic flow demands different poses than a restorative session. Similarly, adapting pose sequences for varying experience levels is fundamental to crafting an accessible and nurturing class environment.

The structure of a session is akin to crafting a story, with an introduction, climax, and resolution. The warm-up opens the narrative, poses build the plot, and the cooldown offers the conclusion. Each chapter of this story flows seamlessly into the next, with transitions as crucial as the poses themselves, weaving a tapestry of continuous movement.

Ultimately, a supremely prepared class is as immersive and empowering as it is educational. It's not about rigidly adhering to a set plan; it's weaving a flexible framework that anticipates the dynamic nature of a group practice. This approach fosters a learning environment that encourages exploration and growth, emboldening students to stretch their boundaries, both physically and mentally.

Effective preparation combines knowledge, anticipation, and adaptability to lay the groundwork for an impactful yoga class.

Center Yourself to Guide Others: The Adaptable Instructor's Blueprint

A yoga instructor's realm is fluid, and preparation serves as both anchor and compass. We must strike a balance between meticulous planning and the capacity to navigate the ebbs and flows of an actual class.

The Balanced Flow Framework

This process, our Balanced Flow Framework, sets forth an adaptable path that embraces the planned while welcoming the spontaneous. It has an ultimate goal: empowered teaching that can pivot with poise to the needs of the moment.

Step 1: Preparing for Class Structure and Content

Allocating around 30 minutes to this step is usually needed. Starting with the goals for the yoga session, we set the narrative. What are we aiming at—a story of strength, a tale of tranquility? The plot unfolds with pose selection and breathwork; think of this as casting characters for a play, each with a role that contributes to the overarching theme.

Step 2: Creating Class Materials and Props

About 20 minutes should be dedicated here to muster one's arsenal of tools. Charts, cue cards, and props are the set pieces of our play, enhancing the experience and offering support.

Step 3: Setting the Tone and Atmosphere

Spend 10 minutes to tune the environment for the opening scene. The introduction sets the mood, inviting participants to close their eyes and attune to their breath, akin to a gentle prelude whispering through a concert hall before the symphony's first note.

Step 4: Delivering Instructions and Cues

A planned 5 minutes per instructional set is recommended.

Here we paint with words, guide with gestures, and narrate each sequence. Clarity is the brush, and modifications are the palette through which we ensure each student finds their expression within the poses.

Step 5: Being Present and Adaptable

This final step is ongoing throughout the class. We remain deeply rooted in the present, attentive to the room's energy as a sailor is to the sea. If the current shifts, we adjust our sails, sometimes altering our pre-scored music to better harmonize with the ensemble's rhythm. The class concludes when objectives are met with satisfaction and self-reflection is ignited within the students.

If you could transform rigid plans into fluid action, how might your teaching evolve?

Embodying Authenticity: Teaching from the Heart

Teaching yoga is a practice of transparency, where instructors pour essence into their classes, allowing authenticity to resonate with students. This genuine approach can turn an ordinary class into a sanctuary of self-discovery.

Consider a beacon: steadfast and uniquely shining its light to guide the way. A yoga teacher must be like this light, a beacon of authenticity, illuminating a path not only with skillful teaching but also with the originality of their being. When teachers show up as their genuine selves, they permit their students to do the same, cultivating an atmosphere of trust and inspiration.

Step 1: Preparing for Class Structure and Content

This involves about 30 minutes to chart the course of the class. Here, personal stories and experiences can be weaved into the theme, making the practice more relatable and powerful. Select poses, breathe, and meditations that resonate on a personal level, to share a piece of your journey with your students.

Step 2: Creating Class Materials and Props

Allocate roughly 20 minutes to curate and personalize

your class's materials. Every handout and prop can be an extension of your teaching personality and philosophy.

Step 3: Setting the Tone and Atmosphere

A mere 10 minutes can effectively set the stage, directly reflecting the instructor's style and heart. Through personal anecdotes or thoughtful questions, students are invited to connect deeply with the practice.

Step 4: Delivering Instructions and Cues

Dedicating about 5 minutes per set of instructions, one can balance consistency with the genuine expression. Teach from experience, using language and metaphors that are innately yours, which fosters a deeper teacher-student connection.

Step 5: Being Present and Adaptable

In constant motion throughout the session, being present means being available for connection. This calls for flexibility, not just in the structure but in the very essence of delivery, making each class a unique reflection of the instructor's true self.

The process finds its fulfillment when students leave imbued with a sense of personal connection, empowered in their practice, and reflective of the authenticity they've witnessed.

In unison, preparation, adaptability, and authenticity form the triad that fortifies a yoga teacher's skill, enabling them to guide with confidence and inspire with genuine spirit.

Embrace Your Path to Confident Teaching

As you reach the end of this chapter, it's essential to remember the core principles that pave the way for you to become a confident and impactful yoga instructor. **Preparation, practice, and authenticity** are the pillars that uphold your teaching journey. By diligently crafting your class sequences, honing your teaching skills through regular practice, and infusing your unique self into every session, you create a space where your students can truly flourish.

Trust in Your Preparation

Effective preparation is the scaffolding of a successful yoga class. As you meticulously plan your sequences, consider the flow, theme, and intention behind each practice. Tailor your classes to address the needs of your students while staying true to your authentic teaching style. Remember, preparation is your roadmap to navigate the class smoothly and with confidence.

Embrace Your Authentic Self

Authenticity is the key to connection. Infuse your classes with your genuine self, allowing your personality and passion for yoga to shine through. When you teach from an authentic place, you invite your students to do the same, fostering a space where exploration and growth are encouraged. Embrace who you are, and let that authenticity guide your teaching.

Cultivate Confidence Through Practice

Confidence is not built overnight; it grows with practice. Regularly stepping onto the mat to practice teaching, refining your sequences, and finding your voice as an instructor is crucial. Embrace each opportunity to teach as a chance to learn and grow. Over time, your confidence will naturally flourish as you immerse yourself in the art of teaching.

Step Into Your Teaching Journey

As you blend preparation, practice, and authenticity in your teaching, you set yourself on a path towards becoming a confident and inspiring yoga instructor. Remember, each class is a new opportunity to guide, inspire, and connect with your students. Embrace the process, stay true to yourself, and watch as your teaching journey unfolds with grace and authenticity.

10

Your Companion on the Journey to Teacherhood

Dawn unfurled itself across the small town as Oliver stepped onto the dew-drenched grass, the gentle hum of the waking world accompanying his every move. Inside the modest studio that Oliver called his sanctum, scattered mats lay in wait for the day's transformation they would witness — from mere nylon rectangles on a wooden floor to platforms of potential and enlightenment. This was his temple, his office, his schoolroom; here, Oliver was both student and teacher, drawn to the reflection of his soul in the mirror of his practice.

As the first eager yogis drifted in, a tangle of ambition and apprehension filled Oliver's chest. The book, "Enlighten Your Path," rested heavily in his palm, a reminder of the responsibilities that pressed against his ribs, echoing the beat of his heart. He needed that mix of wisdom and strategy today as he faced his own trepidation — the mounting pressure of guiding this new flock towards the light of knowledge he was still striving to fully grasp himself.

He closed his eyes, a silent conversation blossoming within him. Images unfurled behind his lids: the days he was a fledgling aspirant, toes finding their tentative grip on the edge of the very mats that now awaited the touch of another round of seekers. Would he be able to instill in them the passion, the grace, the strength he had been gifted by his own mentors? Could he be the vessel through which the ancient discipline would whisper its secrets?

The sunrise spilled through the studio windows, casting prisms of light that danced across the room. It painted the faces of the students in hues of gold and amber — warriors ready for battle, though their war was against the confines of their own limitations rather than against each other. They each carried their unique stories, their personal battles, embroidered into the fabric of their beings, visible only to those who bothered to look close enough.

As he wove through the tapestry of bodies, adjusting a hip here, straightening a spine there, he recalled a passage: "Your journey will be unique, a blend of the teachings that have shaped you and the personal flavor you bring to the mat each day." It was his mantra, a chant that played with each breath he guided, each stretch he facilitated, each moment of understanding he shared. He would shape their paths as his was shaped — with care, with respect, with love.

The session ended, and as the room emptied, Oliver sat with his back to the studio's aged oak door, the book now open in his lap. Light danced upon the pages, inviting him into its depths. In silent contemplation, he pondered the paths that had brought each student to his door. 'Could he be the one to light the way, or was he merely a stepping stone on their journey?'

A Voyage of Transformative Wisdom

As you stand at the brink of completing your yoga teacher training, you are poised to leap from the rooted foundation of study to the expansive freedom of teaching. Your journey has been paved with the enlightenment of ancient practices and the personal growth that comes with deeply understanding them. At its core, becoming a yoga instructor is about more than simply mastering a set of poses; it's about awakening the spirit of guidance within you. You are about to join a lineage of teachers whose shared mission is to better the world one asana at a time.

The chapters thus far have equipped you with comprehensive strategies, skills, and practices vital to your growth as an instructor. Yet, this near-final chapter, "Your Companion on the Journey to Teacherhood," aims to solidify that wisdom, offering perspective as you inch closer to the coveted role of a yoga teacher. Here, we will **leverage the guide** you hold in your hands through the complex tapestry of yoga teacher training, ensuring no thread is left unexamined.

Your education has been steeped in tradition, anatomy, philosophy, and the sheer physicality of yoga. However, the true metamorphosis occurs when you apply this knowledge to teaching others. In this chapter, we stress the importance of **embracing personal growth** and pursuing excellence. As you internalize the teachings, each page becomes a reflection of your evolution from student to teacher. The wisdom captured here is meant to serve not just as knowledge to be recalled, but as an integral part of your being.

Embarking on this transformative journey requires courage and an open heart. You must be prepared to **shape your unique path** into the world of yoga instruction, keeping in mind that the journey does not end once the training is complete. This journey is ongoing, and this guide is designed to be revisited as you evolve, facing new challenges and celebrating new accomplishments.

The core problem this guide addresses is the overwhelming scope of study that can often intimidate the budding yoga instructor. It serves to distill vast and varied knowledge into digestible elements, crafting a learning experience that is both informative and manageable. As we meld the practical with the philosophical, this chapter, in particular, highlights the transitional phase where learning curves bend towards teaching opportunities.

The end result of your engagement with this guide is a calm confidence as you prepare to teach your first class. You have been armed with a wealth of knowledge — from understanding the nuances of alignment to engaging students with empathy. But now is the time to look inwardly and outwardly to cement your identity as a yoga instructor. The strategies and reflections herein are not simply teachings; they are seeds planted for a garden of wisdom that will grow with each class you lead.

Remember, great teachers are not born from the completion of a training program alone; they are nurtured through continuous learning, self-reflection, and the open exchange of knowledge with peers and mentors. As you step forward, using this guide as your compass, know that each day presents an opportunity to refine your craft and to enlighten not just your path but the paths of those you will guide.

Let the momentum of your training propel you into the world of teaching with grace and resilience. Align your intentions with the practices you share, and see each teaching moment as a thread in the beautiful tapestry of your yoga journey. The interconnectedness of your experience is not merely with the poses but with the hearts and minds of your students. As this chapter closes, the practice of teaching truly begins, affirming the notion that enlightenment is not a state to reach but a path to walk — tirelessly and blissfully.

Leverage the Guide Through Yoga Teacher Training

Imagine you've just received a well-worn map from an experienced traveler. It's not just any map; it's a treasure trove of wisdom, filled with notations, tips, and secrets. "Enlighten Your Path" shares similarities with this precious map, serving as your navigational tool through the rich landscape of yoga teacher training. As you unfurl its pages, like the corners of the map, it begins to reveal the intricacies and nuances necessary to steer you through your journey.

The guide is structured smartly, anticipating the hurdles

and questions that come alive in the minds of aspiring instructors. Sections are dedicated to in-depth explorations of yogic philosophy, anatomy, and the delicate art of sequencing. Like signposts on a trail, each chapter highlights crucial landmarks in the yoga teacher's voyage, from mastering the foundational postures to crafting a resonant voice that serves both beginners and seasoned practitioners.

As you delve into the art of teaching yoga, the guide becomes a silent mentor. You learn not only how to execute and instruct poses but also how to embed your classes with the kind of inspiration that touches students profoundly. It breathes life into the technical aspects, such as modifying postures for different bodies, and weaves in the soft skills, like active listening and empathy, which make a yoga teacher truly exceptional.

Yet this guide does more than instruct; it encourages self-reflection and growth. Each lesson is not just a step on a path but a mirror held up to your inner growth, challenging you to expand beyond your perceived limits. The analogy here is simple: just as a seed requires the right conditions to sprout, an aspiring yoga instructor needs the proper guidance to grow. The pages of "Enlighten Your Path" offer that nurturing environment where knowledge and self-awareness bloom.

Let this guide be your compass, turning the complexity of teacher training into a journey of clarity and confidence.

Embrace Personal Growth

As we turn the pages of understanding, we notice that learning is an individual experience. Your growth as a teacher will not mirror that of another, and the wisdom within these pages serves as a reservoir from which you can draw your unique form of inspiration and strength. Every chapter serves as a palette for your self-improvement and the pursuit of excellence.

The pursuit of excellence is, fundamentally, a personal commitment to elevating oneself continuously. It's about honing your skills, deepening your knowledge, and nourishing your spirit. Just as a gardener tirelessly tends to soil and plants to cultivate a bountiful garden, you, too, must tend to the garden of your practice with patience and care to reap the fruits of excellence.

But personal growth in yoga extends beyond the mat and the classroom. It infuses your daily interactions and the quiet moments of reflection. It's the fortitude to hold a difficult pose, and it's equally the courage to face life's challenges with equanimity. The wisdom in this guide doesn't just fill your cup; it transforms you into a vessel, steadily pouring insights into all areas of your life.

It's crucial, however, to remember that personal growth often feels like an expansive, sometimes uncomfortable stretch, much like the first time you glide into Pigeon pose. Growth can tug at the tight, untouched fibers of your being, urging you to explore depths within yourself previously uncharted. The discomfort, though, is a sign of impending transformation - a natural byproduct of stepping into grander versions of oneself.

Let these analogies serve not to define but to illustrate the personal evolution awaiting you. Each step taken is a deliberate act of self-betterment, and each insight gained is a testament to your dedication.

Could your commitment to growth on the mat be the key to unlocking your potential beyond it?

Set Forth on a Transformative Journey

Setting foot on the path to becoming a yoga instructor is akin to planting a garden. You start with a parcel of land - your inherent talents and passion for yoga - and with the right tools and knowledge, you begin to cultivate it. "Enlighten Your Path" serves as a comprehensive guide, from planting the seeds to nurturing full growth, shaping a practice that is distinctively yours.

In this transformative journey, facts are your seeds. As you read through sections detailing alignment, breathing techniques, and the history of yoga, you are sowing the foundation of your garden. With each new concept mastered, you nurture these seeds with the water of practice and the soil of experience.

But facts alone don't create a teacher; it is the spirit with which you teach that breathes life into the lessons. Your unique path as an instructor is the trellis upon which the vine of your teaching style grows. It twists and turns, shaped by personal experiences, beliefs, and the wisdom you gain from both successes and setbacks.

Imagine each class as an authentic expression, a single bloom in the rich tapestry of your teaching garden. No class is exactly like another - each comes with its own colors, fragrances, and textures. The guide encourages you to embrace your authenticity, to let your individuality shine through the poses and the pauses, creating an experience that resonates with your students.

Remember, transformation is not an event but a process. As you continue to grow and shape your path with each turn of the page, you become more attuned to the subtleties of teaching, the intricate dance of guiding others, and the joy of witnessing evolution - both your own and that of your students.

As we connect the dots between guiding wisely, embracing growth, and shaping a unique path, let "Enlighten Your Path" be your steadfast ally on this transformative journey.

Embrace the Journey Ahead

As you reach the end of this chapter, reflect on the transformative journey you are about to embark on as a yoga instructor. **"Enlighten Your Path"** has equipped you with the tools, insights, and encouragement needed to navigate the intricate world of teacher training. Remember, this book is not just a manual; it is your companion, guiding you through the challenges and triumphs that lie ahead.

Trust in Your Growth

Now is the time to embrace personal growth and the pursuit of excellence as you absorb the wisdom within these pages. Every word you've read, every concept you've grasped, has prepared you for the rewarding path of becoming a yoga instructor. **Trust in your abilities** to assimilate this knowledge and let it flourish within you.

Shape Your Unique Path

As you close this chapter and the book as a whole, set forth on your transformative journey using the guide to shape your unique path as a yoga instructor and beyond. **Apply the strategies, skills, and encouragement provided** in **"Enlighten Your Path"** to not just become a yoga teacher, but to become the best version of yourself.

In the vast landscape of yoga instruction, you now hold the compass. Let it guide you through the uncertainties, the doubts, and the challenges, knowing that every step you take is a step towards fulfilling your dream. Your journey to teacherhood starts now. Take a deep breath, step confidently onto the path, and embrace the light within you as you share the gift of yoga with the world.

Embarking On Your Yoga Journey: A Foundation for Future Growth

As we reach the conclusion of this enriching journey together, it's essential to reflect on the essence of what we've shared and uncovered. The path to becoming a yoga instructor is sprinkled with challenges, joys, endless learning, and, most importantly, self-discovery. Remember, mastering the art of yoga instruction is more than acquiring knowledge; it's about embracing a lifestyle, a philosophy, and a commitment to personal growth and well-being.

Bringing Your Practice into the Real World

The teachings in these pages are designed to translate seamlessly into your daily practices and teaching methodologies. From the Sanskrit terms that seemed like a foreign language to the intricate anatomy that appeared daunting at first, each concept has been a stepping stone preparing you for this moment. As you stand at the threshold of your teaching career, consider how you can weave these lessons into the tapestry of your classes, ensuring each student's experience is transformative.

Incorporate storytelling to bring ancient philosophies to life. Imagine using the epic tales of the Bhagavad Gita to illustrate the principles of karma yoga, making the concept accessible and engaging for your students.

Use analogies and metaphors when explaining complex postures or breathing techniques. Just as the lotus flower rises through muddy waters to blossom, remind your students that strength and beauty often emerge from facing challenges.

Recapitulating the Essence of Our Journey

We've traversed through the essential groundwork necessary for a fulfilling transition into teacherhood - from the history and philosophy of yoga, understanding the physical and spiritual anatomy, to the intricate dance of managing a classroom and forming a personal teaching style. Each chapter was meticulously crafted to build your confidence and ensure that the knowledge you carry forward is both profound and practical.

At the heart of this journey has been the encouragement to cultivate a **deep personal practice**—the true wellspring of your teaching. Remember, the most impactful instructors teach from a place of authenticity and personal experience.

Guidance for the Road Ahead

Harness the insights gained from this book by starting small. Perhaps, initiate a community class in a local park, offering a safe space for others to explore their yoga practice under your guidance. Take every opportunity to teach, learn, and evolve. Your development as a teacher is perpetual, growing with each class you conduct and every student you mentor.

Acknowledge that the path of learning is infinite. The areas we've explored represent the foundational layers upon which you can build a vibrant tapestry of knowledge and experience. Continuing your education, be it through workshops, advanced certifications, or personal study, is crucial for your evolution as an instructor and as an individual.

Taking the Leap

Now, it is time for action. Let this book serve as your initial guidepost, but know that the real learning comes through practice, making mistakes, and finding your unique voice. Embrace the uncertainties and the joys that come with being a beginner again. Trust in the process and believe in the value you bring as a yoga instructor.

May you move forward with confidence, humility, and the eagerness to share the gift of yoga with the world.

And as you embark on this noble path, remember the words of T.K.V. Desikachar:

"The success of Yoga does not lie in the ability to perform postures but in how it positively changes the way we live our life and our relationships."

Your journey has just begun, and the world awaits the unique light you are ready to shine. Namaste.

www.ingramcontent.com/pod-product-compliance
Lightning Source LLC
Chambersburg PA
CBHW060513280326
41933CB00014B/2949